THE HEALING DIVERTICULITIS COOKBOOK

THE HEALING
DIVERTICULITIS
COOKBOOK

Recipes to Soothe Inflammation and Relieve Symptoms

TERRI WARD, MS, FNTP, CGP

PHOTOGRAPHY BY DARREN MUIR

ROCKRIDGE
PRESS

Copyright © 2022 by Rockridge Press

All rights reserved. No part of this publication may be reproduced, stored in a retrieval system, or transmitted in any form or by any means, electronic, mechanical, photocopying, recording, scanning, or otherwise without the prior written permission of the Publisher. Requests to the Publisher for permission should be addressed to the Permissions Department, Rockridge Press, 1955 Broadway, Suite 400, Oakland, CA 94612.

First Rockridge Press trade paperback edition 2022

Rockridge Press and the Rockridge Press logo are trademarks or registered trademarks of Callisto Media Inc. and/or its affiliates in the United States and other countries and may not be used without written permission.

For general information on our other products and services, please contact our Customer Care Department within the United States at (866) 744-2665, or outside the United States at (510) 253-0500.

Paperback ISBN: 978-1-63878-043-4
eBook ISBN: 978-1-63878-240-7

Manufactured in the United States of America

Interior and Cover Designer: Amanda Kirk
Art Producer: Maya Melenchuk
Editor: Rachelle Cihonski
Production Editor: Rachel Taenzler
Production Manager: Martin Worthington

Photography © 2022 Darren Muir

Cover image: Turkey Albondigas Soup, page 51

10 9 8 7 6 5 4 3 2 1 0

*I dedicate this book to
my loved ones and others
with diverticular disease.
I hope these tools and resources
help you heal and thrive.*

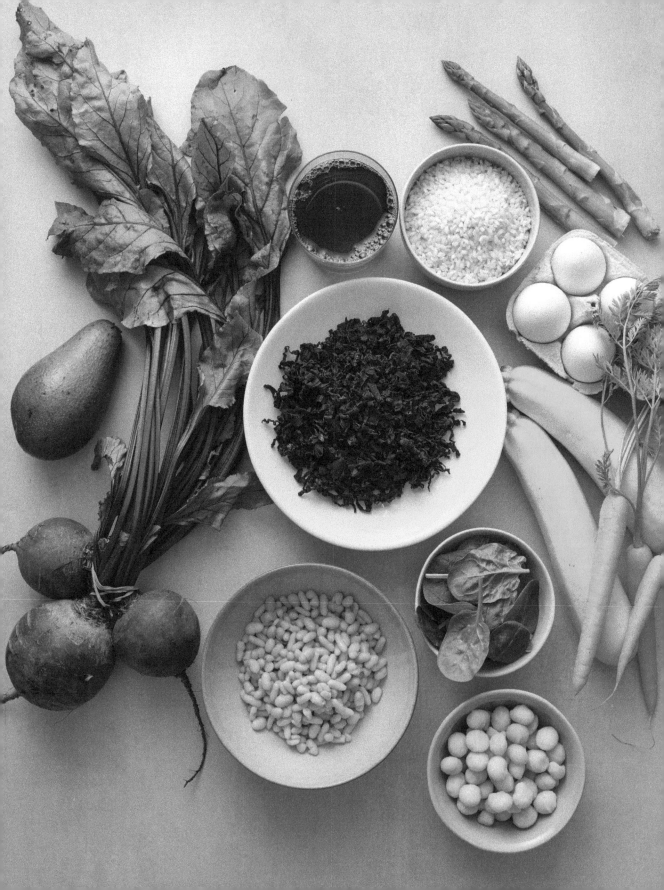

CONTENTS

INTRODUCTION

iverticulitis is a challenging and personal disease. Getting food on the table is hard enough as it is, but if you're in pain, not feeling well, and/or anxious about which foods might trigger a flare-up, it can seem impossible. If you're feeling confused or frustrated about not knowing what's safe to eat or do not have the support and resources you need to implement a diverticulitis diet, I get it. If this sounds like you, this dietary guide and cookbook was written for you.

I'm Terri Ward, and I'm a recovering certified public accountant. After many "taxing" years as a CPA, my health was suffering and my passion was waning. My gut was a mess! My pain and inflammation were out of control. I remember standing in the kitchen, crying, one day. My husband asked what was wrong, and I replied, "I'm afraid I'm going to feel like this forever, and you won't understand."

Thankfully, I healed my gut and recovered my health with nutrition and lifestyle changes. Then one day, I had an aha moment. I realized the health issues that caused me to radically change my diet were a blessing, not a curse—that they ultimately made me healthier overall. I knew I had to help others do the same. So, I set out on a mission and went back to school. I earned a master of science degree in Human Nutrition and Functional Medicine and two nutrition certifications.

Now, as a functional nutritionist, I help people create a sustainable plan to heal their guts and take back their health without spending a fortune. Too often, patients leave their doctor's office scared and confused about diverticulitis and other chronic diseases. I help eliminate the confusion and cut years off the struggle of trying to figure things out on your own.

Over the years, I've learned to create recipes and meal plans for lots of different dietary restrictions. I've discovered work-arounds and substitutions that make healthy eating easy. With the most current dietary guidance for all phases of diverticular disease, this book provides what you need to ease your fear and anxiety over diverticulitis, alleviate pain and inflammation, heal your gut, and achieve long-term success. Always check with your health-care practitioner before using the information in this or any health-related book. I'm not a doctor and never advise against following your doctor's advice. My goal here is to show you the most recent information and communicate it in an understandable way—to empower you to make the right decisions and take control of your own health.

Like my website, TerriWard.com, and my Facebook group, Healthy Guts Healthy Temples with Terri Ward, this dietary guide and cookbook provides delicious recipes and tips promoting gut and holistic health. In the following pages, you'll find the resources you need to make healthy eating easy and enjoyable, including what to eat and when, tips for making things easier, sample meal plans, and 80 easy recipes for different stages of diverticular disease.

Let's get started on creating a healthier you!

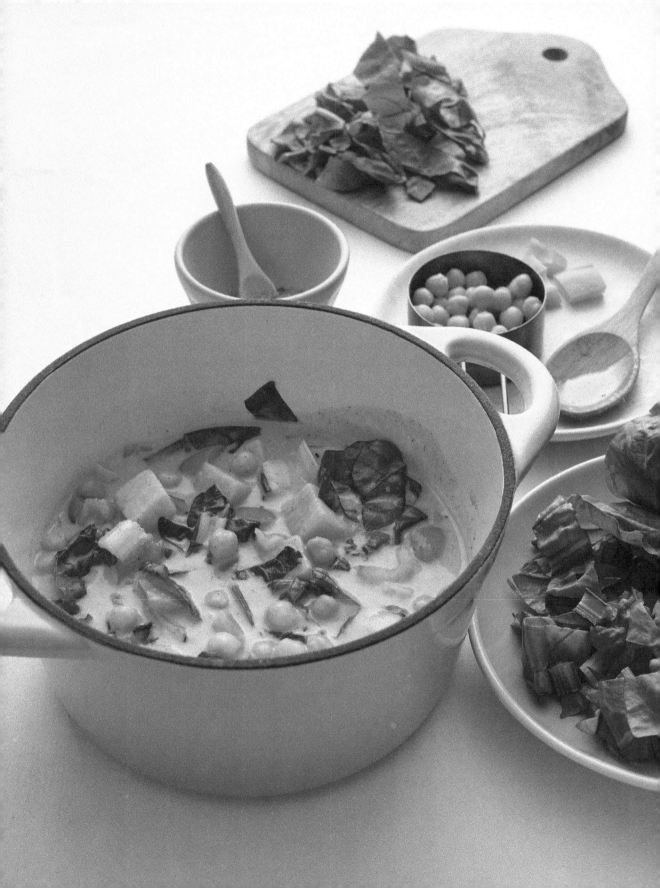

Chapter 1

EATING WITH DIVERTICULAR DISEASE

n this chapter, we'll cover the basics of diverticular disease, including what it is, its causes and risk factors, and treatment. Then we'll take an in-depth look at the diverticulitis diet. I'll explain which foods to eat or avoid, depending on the stage of your disease, and I'll answer some frequently asked questions; discuss digestion, comorbidities, and tips for gut health; and provide meal plans for each stage.

DIVERTICULAR DISEASE: AN OVERVIEW

Diverticulosis is a disease of the large intestine (the colon) in which pouches called diverticula protrude through weak areas in the inner lining of the colon. Diverticulosis is simply *having* these pouches, or diverticula. When the pouches become inflamed or infected, it's called diverticulitis. Diverticular disease includes both diverticulosis and diverticulitis.

Diverticulosis versus Diverticulitis

For most people with diverticulosis, it causes no problems. But for some, symptoms like abdominal tenderness, mild abdominal cramps, swelling or bloating, and/or constipation can develop. For an unfortunate 5 percent, diverticulitis can develop.

Symptoms of diverticulitis include lower abdominal pain and/or cramping, nausea, fever, chills, loss of appetite, constipation or (less commonly) diarrhea, and rectal bleeding. Acute diverticulitis is serious and can be life-threatening, so it's important to seek medical attention promptly.

Risk Factors and Causes

While researchers are still working to understand the causes of and treatments for diverticulitis, know that there are very manageable ways to help ease your symptoms and live a healthy, pain-free life. We can't definitively say any one thing causes diverticular disease, but we now know several related factors that increase your risk of diverticulitis. Let's talk about those risk factors so you can better understand how to prevent flare-ups and complications.

Dysbiosis: Your microbiome is the collection of all microbes, such as bacteria, fungi, viruses, and their genes, which naturally live on and inside your body. Dysbiosis is an imbalance in the types of microbes, generally a reduction in diversity and beneficial bacterial and/or an overgrowth of harmful bacteria. Researchers believe gut microbes play a role in the development of diverticular disease. Genetics, diseases, surgeries, medications, stress, and your diet are some of the factors that influence your microbiome. I recommend working with a practitioner who does stool testing to help balance your unique microbiome.

Altered gut motility and leaky gut: Gut motility is the process of food travelling through your digestive tract. Various studies link altered gut motility to diverticulitis. Slow motility can cause constipation, intestinal inflammation, and leaky gut. When your gut is leaky, things get through the barrier into your bloodstream that shouldn't. When your immune system encounters something foreign, it launches an attack, triggering inflammation.

Inflammation: As with most chronic diseases, inflammation plays a large role in diverticulitis and its complications. Contributors to inflammation include dysbiosis, allergies, autoimmune disease, infection, poor digestion, poor sleep, environmental toxins, stress, and increased insulin. In turn, inflammation can contribute to leaky gut and dysbiosis.

Other risk factors: Smoking, vitamin D deficiency, and certain drugs, including NSAIDs (nonsteroidal anti-inflammatory drug), aspirin, corticosteroids, and opioids.

The good news is most of the risk factors—including those discussed next that cause dysbiosis, altered gut motility, leaky gut, and inflammation—are within your control. Age and genetics are factors outside of your control, but alone, they're not your fate. In fact, four steps you can take right now to reduce your risk are: 1) work with a professional to heal your gut and balance your microbiome; 2) eat a high-fiber, anti-inflammatory diet; 3) exercise and maintain a healthy weight; and 4) manage your stress. Let's explore these steps more closely.

Diet: Most large studies indicate low fiber intake is the main dietary factor relating to diverticulitis. A diet of red and processed meats, refined grains and sugars, and high-fat dairy products with low fiber intake is highly inflammatory. Some studies show an association between eating red meat and a higher risk for diverticular disease, colon cancer, and obesity. Drinking alcohol is also associated with diverticular bleeding and can alter your microbial balance and cause leaky gut, leading to inflammation in the gut and elsewhere in your body.

Obesity and/or lack of exercise: Obesity is a risk factor for many digestive disorders, including diverticulitis, while regular exercise is associated with a reduced risk of diverticulitis. The American Gastroenterological Association's guidelines recommend healthy adults get at least 90 minutes of vigorous activity every week. Regular exercise helps balance your microbiome, making it more anti-inflammatory. It also helps reduce stress, fatigue, bloating, and constipation.

Stress: Stress plays a role in gut motility and your weight. It also contributes to leaky gut and promotes inflammatory gut microbes, which starts an inflammatory cascade that can lead to infection.

Complications

When bacteria get stuck in a pouch, an infection can occur and spread to other diverticula, leading to complications. Complications of diverticular disease can be life-threatening and generally demand immediate medical attention. These complications include:

Bleeding: The result of ruptured blood vessels. Most often, bleeding will stop on its own and has no associated pain. In some cases, treatment or surgery is needed.

Perforation: A tiny hole or tear in the colon that allows its contents to leak into the abdomen.

Abscess: A collection of pus in a specific place or part of the body surrounded by inflamed tissue. If antibiotic treatment doesn't work, surgery or a draining procedure may be required.

Peritonitis: Inflammation of the peritoneum, the tissue lining the inner wall of the abdomen and covering most of the abdominal organs. If a large abscess ruptures and spreads to the peritoneum, immediate surgery is needed to clean the infection and prevent sepsis, a systemic infection that is potentially life-threatening.

Stricture or obstruction: A narrowing or blockage in the colon caused by scar tissue from a prior infection. Partial obstructions sometimes clear on their own, but if you cannot pass stool, surgery may be required.

Fistula: An abnormal connection between an organ and another structure. In diverticular disease, a tunnel may form between the colon and the small intestine, bladder, skin, or vagina. Surgery may be necessary to remove the fistula and the affected part of the colon.

Treatment

For many who suffer with diverticulitis, optimal care seems elusive. Different treatment strategies are required for each stage of the disease, and because everyone is different, a personalized approach is needed.

Conventional medical treatments include:

- Fiber for preventing recurrence of flare-ups or development of complications

- Rest, antibiotics, and pain control for flare-ups

- Surgery for selected cases

Antibiotics are prescribed routinely for acute diverticulitis, sometimes repeatedly, and can cause adverse effects and allergic reactions. One of the commonly used antibiotics for diverticulitis has a black box warning for serious risks. The additional risk of antibiotic resistance and adverse effects on the microbiome are concerning. I recommend you research all medications you're prescribed and talk to your practitioner or pharmacist about your options. Also see Frequently Asked Questions (page 6) for more information.

I recommend augmenting your treatment with some proactive gut healing to prevent recurrences and the need for repeated antibiotics. A proactive functional medicine (root cause) approach would address *your* personal risk factors and underlying conditions. Diet, supplementation, and lifestyle changes would tackle dysbiosis, leaky gut, inflammation, stress, and gut motility.

FREQUENTLY ASKED QUESTIONS

Q Can I drink alcohol?
Alcohol is inflammatory and can irritate your intestinal lining. It can also affect gut motility and interact with medications you're taking. After healing, some people can add back moderate amounts when they consume about twice as much water with the alcohol. Check with your practitioner after your symptoms resolve.

Q Can I drink coffee or tea?
Besides caffeine, coffee contains additional compounds that can stimulate bowel movements in some, but not all people. Coffee and some teas are acidic, which can irritate your stomach. If the acid bothers you, or if you have IBS-D or antibiotic-induced diarrhea, you may want to switch to herbal tea in the morning. Talk to your practitioner and check the ingredients of anything you're adding to your coffee.

Q Can I drink carbonated beverages?
Drinking carbonated beverages can cause gas and bloating, which can lead to increased pressure and abdominal pain. It can also cause loss of bone density and problems upstream in the digestive tract. For these reasons and because carbonated beverages generally contain unhealthy ingredients, they are best avoided.

Q Are antibiotics always necessary?
Recent research indicates that for mild, uncomplicated diverticulitis, antibiotics do not shorten the recovery period, nor do they influence the need for surgery or prevent complications. A study published in the *Journal of the Royal Society of Medicine* revealed it takes 17 years for new science to be incorporated into clinical practice. Thus, I recommend sharing and discussing with your practitioner the clinical trials by Chabok et al. and Daniels et al. listed in the References (see page 133).

Q **Do I need to have a colonoscopy after a flare-up?**
Doctors like to do colonoscopies after flare-ups so they can get in and see what's going on. A colonoscopy can help exclude colon cancer or other diagnoses. Discuss this with your doctor.

Q **Will I need surgery?**
Surgery to remove the affected part of the colon is decided on a case-by-case basis. It's indicated for immunocompromised patients, perforations, fistulas, strictures, abscesses that can't be drained effectively, and cases that don't respond to IV antibiotics. Someone who's had multiple attacks may choose surgery to prevent future attacks.

Q **Are nutritional deficiencies a concern?**
Most nutrient absorption occurs in the small intestine, but gut microbes in the colon produce biotin; vitamins B_6, B_{12}, and K; and short-chain fatty acids (SCFAs). The SCFA butyrate is especially important for helping prevent leaky gut, combatting inflammation, protecting the brain, and reducing colon cancer risk. You can take butyrate supplements, but it's best obtained by eating butter from grass-fed cows and eating prebiotic foods like chickpeas, apples, garlic, and almonds that feed butyrate-producing bacteria.

Q **What is the best fiber supplement?**
The best fiber for diverticular disease comes from fruits, vegetables, and some grains. These foods are also good sources of antioxidants and flavonoids, which enhance tissue integrity, proving more beneficial than just fiber. Metamucil is frequently recommended, but I'm not a fan of artificial flavors and colors. The main ingredient, psyllium husk, which I often use in smoothies and baked goods, can be purchased separately (see Resources, page 130).

THE ROLE OF DIET

Everything that enters your digestive tract or gut affects everything below it. Since diverticulitis involves inflammation, eating inflammatory foods like gluten, dairy, soy, sugar, artificial sweeteners, caffeine, processed and refined foods, fried foods, food additives, MSG, and alcohol should be avoided. Other foods may be inflammatory or trigger foods for you; those foods should be avoided as well.

When inflammation or infection strikes, it's important not to irritate your digestive tract with food so that it can heal. The three dietary steps for healing after a flare-up involve: 1) a few days of clear liquids only during a flare-up; 2) two or more weeks of low-fiber foods to recover from a flare-up; and 3) high-fiber maintenance to prevent flare-ups. In the first two phases, you'll eat smaller amounts frequently throughout the day to ensure you get enough calories without overeating. Consult your practitioner on the timing. Move slowly through each phase, adding different foods slowly, and closely monitor your symptoms using a food journal (see page 128).

This diet is not a high-fat keto diet, but it's also not a low-fat diet. Our bodies use fat for energy, brain health, cell membranes, producing hormones, and absorbing fat-soluble vitamins. They just need the right fats from whole-food sources like avocados, olive oil, nuts, seeds, and fatty fish. Butter, ghee, and coconut oil are healthy in moderation, but trans fats, hydrogenated or partially hydrogenated oils, and refined vegetable oils should be avoided.

CONSIDERING COMMON COMORBIDITIES

Some of the risk factors discussed earlier can be considered comorbidities because they commonly coexist with diverticulitis. Coronary heart disease and chronic kidney disease, as well as high blood pressure, cholesterol, and high uric acid, all increase the risk of diverticular bleeding.

All these conditions as well as the following ones can be improved with the diet and lifestyle changes discussed in this book. The recipes in this book are designed with these common comorbidities in mind, and adjustments to support these conditions are noted here or in the recipes. For example, feel free to substitute egg whites for whole eggs as needed to support your own health goals and needs.

IBS: Irritable bowel syndrome is common among those with diverticulitis. Most IBS is caused by SIBO (small intestinal bacterial overgrowth). A low-FODMAP diet, which eliminates certain sugars that can cause intestinal distress, is often recommended for IBS and SIBO. This isn't a low-FODMAP cookbook, but many of the recipes are low-FODMAP. For example, I've used Garlic Oil (page 115) rather than garlic and only the green parts of scallions and leeks in the recipes.

Hypertension (high blood pressure): If you have salt sensitivity, you can reduce or eliminate the salt in recipes in the High-Fiber Phase. Do not omit salt in the Clear Liquid or Low-Fiber Phases. Salt provides sodium, which is important as an electrolyte and for keeping you hydrated. Always use pink Himalayan salt or unrefined sea salt rather than table salt.

Type 2 Diabetes: All phases of this diet can be safe with diabetes, and the High-Fiber Phase should help lower your blood sugar. Other dietary or medication changes may be needed, so stay in communication with the practitioner who manages your diabetes.

DURING A FLARE-UP: CLEAR LIQUID PHASE

When diverticulosis causes symptoms, it's called a diverticulitis attack or flare-up. When the symptoms are severe, your body can't tolerate solid foods, so a clear liquid diet is recommended. A clear liquid diet keeps your intestines clear to avoid straining your digestive system. In other words, you stay hydrated while your bowels rest and heal.

You won't get sufficient calories and nutrients in this phase, so it's only recommended for a few days or until your symptoms are less severe. Drinking nutritious fluids like chicken or beef bone broth, vegetable broth, and coconut water will help keep your electrolyte levels balanced.

Many electrolyte drinks and powders are loaded with sugars, colors, and other undesirable additives. In the Resources section, I've listed some healthier "clean" versions and electrolyte drops you can put in your juice or other drinks (see page 130). In the electrolyte recipes, I recommend Himalayan pink salt for its trace mineral content and flavor. In the other recipes, you can use either pink salt or sea salt.

Check with your practitioner regarding when to add low-fiber foods. The following chart clarifies what a "clear" liquid is.

EAT THIS	AVOID THAT
Water (plain or flavored), coconut water, and clear, fat-free broths	Solid foods of any kind, including soup with food particles
Coffee or tea with no milk products or creamers	Smoothies, yogurt drinks, sugary or carbonated beverages
Pulp-free fruit juice and ice pops made with juice (apple, berry, cherry, cranberry, grape, pomegranate, etc.)	Citrus, fruit skins, seeds, or pulp
Strained vegetable juice	Milk and milk alternatives, alcohol, tomato juice
Gelatin made with juice or tea	Peanut butter
"Clean" electrolyte drinks	Anything else not in the first column

AFTER A FLARE-UP: LOW-FIBER PHASE

After flare-up symptoms improve, usually within two to four days, you can add 10 to 15 grams of fiber per day to your diet. Your gut is still healing, so to prevent a recurrence, add the fiber slowly, starting with 5 grams or less, to see how your body reacts. Avoid the foods listed in the "Avoid That" column on page 12, as well as any personal trigger foods. You might be hungry, but this is not a time to cheat since this could trigger another flare-up and create a vicious circle.

The goals in this phase are fewer, smaller bowel movements while your gut heals and to ease symptoms like diarrhea, bloating, gas, and stomach cramping. You need to have bowel movements! If you're not having bowel movements, make sure you're drinking enough water and consider adding a little more fiber or taking some magnesium (see Resources, page 130).

The length of this phase depends on you. Your symptoms may take several weeks to resolve before you transition to the High-Fiber Phase. The sooner, the better, but partner with your practitioner about the timing. If you're losing weight, be sure you're getting 0.36 grams of protein per pound of body weight daily to prevent muscle wasting. Please don't get stuck in this phase! Eating refined grains and only 10 to 15 grams of fiber contributes to diverticulitis and other chronic diseases. Seek professional help if you're getting stuck.

In this phase, your food should be soft enough to easily mash with a fork. Go slow, don't overeat, drink lots of water, keep a food journal (see page 128) to learn your trigger foods, and follow the chart on page 12.

	EAT THIS	AVOID THAT
ANIMAL PROTEINS	Tender, lean, and well-cooked, baked, broiled, grilled, or stewed poultry and fish; scrambled, soft-boiled, or poached eggs	Fried meats/poultry/fish/eggs; fatty and gristly meat; rubbery seafood, such as shrimp; tough skins; smoked or cured deli meat; sausage, bacon, and hot dogs
VEGETABLES	Well-cooked, fresh, or canned, without peels, seeds, or stalks: asparagus tips, beets, eggplant, green or wax beans, carrots, potatoes (without skins); pumpkin, rutabaga, tomato sauce (no seeds), spinach, winter squash, yellow squash, zucchini	Legumes; beans; lentils; onions; tofu; raw or undercooked vegetables and certain cooked vegetables: broccoli, Brussels sprouts, cabbage, cauliflower, collard greens, corn, cucumber, green peas, kale, lettuce, okra, highly seasoned or fried potatoes or potato chips, turnips
GRAINS	White bread, biscuits, and plain crackers (no seeds); tortillas; cooked cereals; white rice; noodles; rice pasta; pretzels	Products made from whole grains, including barley, bran, brown rice, bulgur, corn bread, oats, popcorn, quinoa, rye, wheat
FRUITS	Ripe avocados or bananas; soft cantaloupe or honeydew; canned or cooked fruits (no skin or seeds) like applesauce, canned apricots, peaches or pears in juice	Raw or dried fruits, coconut meat, pineapple
DAIRY AND DAIRY ALTERNATIVES	Almond, macadamia nut, or coconut milk; puddings and ice cream made with these	Milk and milk products from cows or goats
BEVERAGES	Coffee, tea, pulp-free juice, strained vegetable juices	Fruit juices with pulp or seeds, prune juice, pear nectar, V8 juice, sugary or carbonated beverages
CONDIMENTS, DRESSINGS, SEASONINGS, ETC.	Ketchup, mayonnaise, mustard, olive oil, coconut oil, gravy, smooth nut and seed butters, honey, molasses, mild herbs and flavorings, lemon juice	Acidic foods and dressings; strongly flavored/spicy seasonings, including black and red pepper, garlic, horseradish, whole-grain mustard, pickles, and relish; sauerkraut; whole seeds or nuts; crunchy nut and seed butters

MAINTENANCE: HIGH-FIBER PHASE

As in the Low-Fiber Phase, you'll want to add fiber slowly until you reach your recommended daily intake (see page 14). Be sure to drink plenty of water and move your body. This is the varied diet with minimal restrictions that you'll want to be on all the time to optimize digestion and combat inflammation.

Keep in mind that there is no snacking in this phase. Your migrating motor complex (MMC) needs to do its job of sweeping out leftover food particles from the small intestine. The MMC isn't triggered while you're digesting food. Spacing meals out at least three to four hours allows the MMC to sweep out food particles, reducing the chance of constipation and bacterial overgrowth.

If you have comorbidities, consult the information on comorbidities earlier in this chapter (see page 9) and partner with your practitioner(s) to come up with a personalized diet and exercise plan.

	EAT THIS	AVOID THAT*
ANIMAL PROTEINS	Baked, broiled, grilled, steamed, or stewed poultry and fish; eggs (rarely red meat)	Fried meats/poultry/fish/eggs; processed and grain-fed meats
DAIRY AND DAIRY ALTERNATIVES	Butter; ghee; yogurt**; almond, macadamia nut, or coconut milk	Most other dairy products
GRAINS	Whole gluten-free grains: brown rice, buckwheat, corn**, millet, oats/oatmeal (gluten-free), popcorn**, quinoa, sorghum, teff, wild rice	Refined grains, processed foods, gluten-containing grains: wheat, barley, rye, and contaminated oats
FRUITS AND VEGETABLES	Fresh, frozen, or lightly cooked fruits, berries, and vegetables	Sweetened fruits, fried vegetables
OTHER	Legumes, nuts, seeds, nut and seed butters, condiments, gluten-free tamari, coconut aminos, olive oil, coconut oil, avocado oil	Refined sugars; corn syrups; sauces with sugar, cream, or gluten; soy sauce; vegetable oils; MSG; preservatives; more than 2 alcoholic drinks daily; artificial sweeteners, colors, and flavors

*These items are generally unhealthy and/or inflammatory.
**Eat these items if tolerated.

Recommended Fiber and Water Intake

Fiber and water work together to form a bulky stool that's easily eliminated. Without sufficient water, fiber can cause constipation.

A recommended fiber intake is 14 grams per 1,000 calories of food. Recognizing that men typically require more calories and older adults require fewer, the charts that follow show recommendations based on gender and age.

RECOMMENDED FIBER INTAKE:

Men ages 19 to 50: 38 grams per day
Men ages 50+: 30 grams per day
Women ages 19 to 50: 25 grams per day
Women ages 50+: 21 grams per day

RECOMMENDED WATER INTAKE:

Men ages 19+: 12 cups (about 3 liters) per day
Women ages 19+: 9 cups (about 2.1 liters) per day

Water is best, but juice, milk, soups, coffee, tea, and herbal teas contribute to your liquid intake. Warm water may be more comforting to your digestive system than cold water.

Eating a Balanced Plate

When you're not experiencing a flare-up or recovering from one, you should strive to eat a balanced diet with lots of color and variety. Eating a variety of different-colored foods from different food groups provides a wide range of:

- Macronutrients (protein, carbohydrates, and fat)

- Micronutrients (vitamins and minerals)

- Phytonutrients (natural plant compounds that promote health and contain antioxidants, generally represented by color)

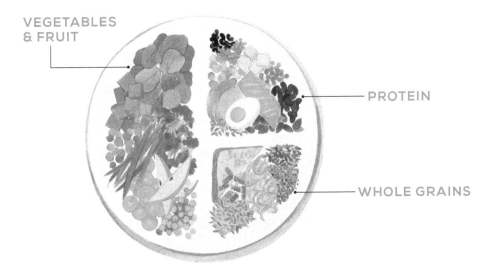

VEGETABLES & FRUIT

PROTEIN

WHOLE GRAINS

You don't have to count calories or calculate macronutrient ratios if you aim for balance on your plate. A balanced high-fiber plate should be at least half fruits and vegetables (mostly vegetables), one-quarter high-fiber starchy vegetables or whole grains, and one-quarter lean protein. An example might be: 4 ounces of chicken breast, ½ cup of cooked brown rice, and 2 cups of steamed vegetables or 1½ cups of vegetables and ½ cup of fruit.

SUPPLEMENTS AND PROBIOTICS

Nutrients are best obtained from the foods we eat, and in a perfect world, those foods would be sufficient. In the real world of depleted soils, fewer plant species, toxic exposures, chronic stress, and sedentary lifestyles, even a balanced, organic diet likely won't provide everything you need.

There is a science to supplementation, so I recommend working with a practitioner to help determine your individual needs and the right forms and doses for you, as well as professional-grade supplements to ensure quality, potency, and bioavailability. It is important to purchase supplements from trusted sources. Your practitioner should know all drugs you're taking to avoid potential interactions.

Probiotics: There's evidence to support using probiotics in diverticular disease to alleviate dysbiosis, leaky gut, and/or inflammation. It's important to use the right strain, however. The effects of probiotics are strain-specific and cannot be conferred by other strains of the same species.

Prebiotics: Your practitioner may also recommend a particular prebiotic depending on which bacteria needs to grow and be fed. The most commonly available prebiotics are fructooligosaccharides (FOS), galactooligosaccharides (GOS), and lactulose.

Fermented foods: Raw (not canned) sauerkraut, kimchi, yogurt, kefir, and other fermented vegetables are an economical source of multiple probiotic strains with other health benefits. Try your own ferment with the easy Fermented Jicama (page 92) recipe.

Supplements: Maintenance supplementation might include a high-quality multivitamin and mineral, vitamin D_3, omega-3 fatty acids (fish oil), and probiotics. Therapeutic supplementation, or taking certain nutrients for a specified purpose for a specified time, may also be beneficial for diverticulitis. Your practitioner's recommendations may include digestive enzymes; gut healing or soothing nutrients, like l-glutamine, marshmallow root, slippery elm, and licorice (DGL); 5-HTP for gut motility; curcumin or CBD for inflammation; and magnesium.

TIPS FOR SUCCESS

Changing your diet and lifestyle is never easy, but neither is being sick and in pain. Eliminating the foods you usually eat is tough, but with some planning and meal prepping, you can have nourishing, safe foods available to reduce temptation.

Meal Planning and Prepping

Meal planning involves planning what you'll eat in advance. Without a plan, you're more likely to eat something you shouldn't.

Meal prepping takes things a step further, to cooking your meals in advance. When I cook, I frequently make extras for refrigerator or freezer leftovers, but when I'm meal prepping, I cook everything I need for the week in one or two days. A couple of hours prepping provides healthy, balanced meals all week to simply reheat. Even if you don't have the time to prep all of the week's meals in advance, batch cooking things like rice or quinoa to have on hand is a great way to cut down on cooking time throughout the week.

Many of the recipes in this book have meal prep and storage guidance to get you started. If you haven't meal prepped before, I recommend starting with just two or three easy recipes. By consolidating cooking tasks and shopping, you'll save a lot of time and get to enjoy some nights off.

Cooking Shortcuts

When you're too tired to cook, consider having a smoothie or breakfast for dinner, like pancakes or scrambled eggs. Keep ingredients on hand for those easy recipes you know and love. Some of my favorite go-to recipes include Tuna Salad with Avocado (page 49) and Turkey-Mayo Roll-Ups (page 88). Almost all the recipes in this book can be made in less time than it would take to drive to a restaurant, order, eat, and drive home. Many of the recipes include shortcut and cooking tips to save you even more time.

Eating Out

Diverticulitis shouldn't ruin your social life. Be prepared to take care of your own needs and use the following tips to eliminate any anxiety over dining away from home.

Tip 1: If you'll be a guest, tell the host you don't expect special accommodations, but for health reasons, you need to know the ingredients in each of the dishes. If the host can't accommodate you, eat only what is obviously safe. If there won't be much you can eat, eat something before you go.

Tip 2: If you're going to a restaurant, check out the menu beforehand. Call ahead and speak with the manager or chef and ask about preparation methods, portion sizes, substitutions, and any unexpected ingredients. Choose a baked, broiled, or grilled protein rather than breaded, battered, or fried, and choose steamed vegetables.

Tip 3: Keep it simple. One of the best meals I've ever had was something basic the chef created based on what I *could* have rather than what I *couldn't* have.

Cravings

Food cravings generally stem from habits, emotions, and brain or body chemistry rather than hunger. Increased cortisol, lack of sleep, low blood sugar, hormonal imbalances, dehydration, and insufficient protein or other nutritional deficiencies may play a role in cravings.

Fortunately, when you start improving your health, you'll shift to a healthier body chemistry. Consider using my Food Reaction Tracker (see page 128) to log your cravings in the mood section. Then, use the results to change your scenario or replace the craving with a healthier alternative when a craving arises.

Your diverticula won't go away, so you'll need to stay proactive about preventing flare-ups. Giving into cravings could trigger a flare-up. If you're confident you've healed, you may be able to indulge once in a great while, but only you can decide if it's worth the risk.

Support

Diverticulitis is a personal disease. Often others aren't comfortable talking about it and/or don't understand the anxiety and concern you have about food. Further, they may think you should just eat more if you're losing weight or that you're lazy or depressed if you're lying around. I get that your life changed with a diagnosis, and I encourage you to find the support and understanding you need. Please don't suffer alone. Consider counseling or joining a support group (in-person or on social media).

SAMPLE MEAL PLANS

In this section, I've provided sample meal plans for each phase of the diverticulitis diet to help you on your healing journey. Each meal plan serves 1 person.

In these meal plans, foods with 5 or more grams of fiber are labeled "high fiber." The labels in the recipe chapters also follow that rule. However, I've included some recipes with 5 or 6 grams of fiber in the low-fiber meal plan and stayed within 10 to 15 grams per day. Likewise, in the High-Fiber Phase, you can, and should, include healthy foods like blueberries and sweet potatoes with fewer than 5 grams of fiber per serving in combination with other foods that help you reach your target (see page 14). Pay attention to how you feel and spread out your target throughout the day.

Flare-Up (3 Days)

The clear liquids will soothe your gut and provide flavor variety. Unless a recipe indicates otherwise, the serving sizes are 1 cup for each of the beverages and broths. If you're hungry and not feeling bloated, you can drink more. Monitor your blood glucose level if you're diabetic. The bone broth cooks for a long time, but none of the recipes require much prep time so you or a caregiver could prep them all in about an hour.

Flare-Up: Clear Liquid Phase (3 Days)

	BREAKFAST	SNACK	LUNCH	SNACK	DINNER
DAY 1	Lemon water Tart Cherry Electrolyte Drink (page 28) Chicken Bone Broth (page 114)	Coffee or tea Cranberry Gelatin (page 100)	Coconut water Beef Bone Broth (page 114, see tip) Ginger tea with honey	Licorice Ice Pops (1) (page 86) Peppermint tea	*Leftover* Chicken Bone Broth Calm magnesium drink (see Resources, page 130)
DAY 2	Lemon water *Leftover* Tart Cherry Electrolyte Drink *Leftover* Beef Bone Broth	Coffee or tea *Leftover* Licorice Ice Pops (1)	Coconut water *Leftover* Chicken Bone Broth Ginger tea with honey	*Leftover* Cranberry Gelatin Peppermint tea	*Leftover* Beef Bone Broth Calm magnesium drink
DAY 3	Lemon water *Leftover* Tart Cherry Electrolyte Drink *Leftover* Chicken Bone Broth	Coffee or tea *Leftover* Cranberry Gelatin	Coconut water *Leftover* Beef Bone Broth Ginger tea with honey	*Leftover* Licorice Ice Pops (1) Peppermint tea	*Leftover* Chicken Bone Broth Calm magnesium drink

Recovery

These next 2 weeks of meals will introduce fiber slowly and minimize your time in the kitchen. Cooking any four or five recipes listed consecutively in one session should require less than an hour of prep time per session.

Recovery: Low-Fiber Phase

WEEK 1	BREAKFAST	SNACK	LUNCH	SNACK	DINNER
SUNDAY	Grape juice (6 ounces) Scrambled egg whites (½ cup)	Pomegranate Electrolyte Drink (page 29)	Creamy Lemon and Rice Soup with Chicken (page 47)	Turkey-Mayo Roll-Ups (page 88)	Easy Chicken and Rice Noodle Soup (page 50)
MONDAY	Grape juice (6 ounces) Scrambled egg whites (½ cup) Canned peaches in juice (½ cup)	*Leftover* Turkey-Mayo Roll-Ups	*Leftover* Easy Chicken and Rice Noodle Soup	*Leftover* Pomegranate Electrolyte Drink	*Leftover* Creamy Lemon and Rice Soup with Chicken
TUESDAY	Creamy Cinnamon-Rice Porridge (page 33)	*Leftover* Pomegranate Electrolyte Drink	*Leftover* Creamy Lemon and Rice Soup with Chicken	*Leftover* Turkey-Mayo Roll-Ups	*Leftover* Chicken and Rice Noodle Soup
WEDNESDAY	*Leftover* Creamy Cinnamon-Rice Porridge ½ ripe banana	Unsweetened applesauce (½ cup)	*Leftover* Easy Chicken and Rice Noodle Soup	Quick Tapioca Pudding (page 106)	*Leftover* Creamy Lemon and Rice Soup with Chicken

continued ▶

Recovery: Low-Fiber Phase *continued*

WEEK 1	BREAKFAST	SNACK	LUNCH	SNACK	DINNER
THURSDAY	*Leftover* Creamy Cinnamon-Rice Porridge ½ ripe banana	Canned peaches in juice (½ cup)	Scalloped Zucchini with Shrimp (page 64)	*Leftover* Quick Tapioca Pudding	Tuna Salad with Avocado (page 49)
FRIDAY	*Leftover* Creamy Cinnamon-Rice Porridge Canned peaches in juice (½ cup)	*Leftover* Quick Tapioca Pudding	*Leftover* Tuna Salad with Avocado	Unsweetened applesauce (½ cup)	*Leftover* Scalloped Zucchini with Shrimp
SATURDAY	Scrambled egg whites (½ cup) Turkey sausage (4 ounces) using Breakfast Sausage Seasoning (page 116) Canned peaches in juice (½ cup)	Unsweetened applesauce (½ cup)	*Leftover* Scalloped Zucchini with Shrimp	*Leftover* Quick Tapioca Pudding	*Leftover* Tuna Salad with Avocado

Recovery: Low-Fiber Phase continued

WEEK 2	BREAKFAST	SNACK	LUNCH	SNACK	DINNER
SUNDAY	Simple Banana Pancakes (page 34) *Leftover* turkey breakfast sausage (4 ounces) *(from Week 1)*	Cran-Apple Electrolyte Slushie (page 30)	Mashed Potatoes with Chicken Gravy (page 66)	Canned peaches in juice (½ cup)	*Leftover* Scalloped Zucchini with Shrimp *(from Week 1)*
MONDAY	*Leftover* Simple Banana Pancakes *Leftover* turkey breakfast sausage (4 ounces) *(from Week 1)*	Soft-boiled egg (1)*	Chicken-Celeriac Soup with Tarragon (page 48)	*Leftover* Cran-Apple Electrolyte Slushie	*Leftover* Mashed Potatoes with Chicken Gravy
TUESDAY	*Leftover* Cran-Apple Electrolyte Slushie Carrot Cake Smoothie (page 40)	Soft-boiled egg (1)*	*Leftover* Mashed Potatoes with Chicken Gravy	Banana Muffins (2) (page 32)	*Leftover* Chicken-Celeriac Soup with Tarragon
WEDNESDAY	Grape juice (6 ounces) *Leftover* Carrot Cake Smoothie	*Leftover* Cran-Apple Electrolyte Slushie	*Leftover* Chicken-Celeriac Soup with Tarragon	Hibiscus-Pomegranate Yogurt Parfait (page 104)	Rice-Crusted Spinach Quiche (page 68)

continued ▶

WEEK 2	BREAKFAST	SNACK	LUNCH	SNACK	DINNER
THURSDAY	Cran-Apple Electrolyte Slushie (page 30) *Leftover* Rice-Crusted Spinach Quiche	*Leftover* Hibiscus-Pomegranate Yogurt Parfait	Turkey Albondigas Soup (page 51)	Unsweetened applesauce (½ cup)	Easy Pumpkin Risotto (page 65)
FRIDAY	Grape juice (6 ounces) *Leftover* Rice-Crusted Spinach Quiche	Unsweetened applesauce (½ cup)	*Leftover* Easy Pumpkin Risotto	*Leftover* Hibiscus-Pomegranate Yogurt Parfait	*Leftover* Turkey Albondigas Soup
SATURDAY	*Leftover* Banana Muffins (2)	*Leftover* Hibiscus-Pomegranate Yogurt Parfait	*Leftover* Rice-Crusted Spinach Quiche	Canned peaches (½ cup)	*Leftover* Easy Pumpkin Risotto

*To soft-boil an egg: Cover the egg with cold water in a saucepan. Bring to a boil over medium-high heat. Lower the heat to a simmer and cook for 5 minutes. Transfer the egg to a colander and run cold water over it to stop the cooking.

Maintenance

This plan slowly increases your fiber up to 25 grams per day. Remember, snacking will prevent your migrating motor complex from doing its job of sweeping out leftover food particles from the small intestine, so avoid snacking. You should be able to get enough rolls (4) and flatbreads (2) from one batch of Grain-Free Baguette, Rolls, or Flatbreads (page 124) to make all the meals this week that serve them. I also suggest batch cooking 3 baked sweet potatoes on Sunday to serve with the Asian-Inspired Turkey Loaf (page 71) and leftovers this week.

Maintenance: High-Fiber Phase

	BREAKFAST	LUNCH	DINNER
SUNDAY	Blueberry-Nut Oatmeal (page 43)	Asian-Inspired Turkey Loaf (page 71) Baked sweet potato (1) (page 71, see tip) Grain-Free Roll (1) (page 124)	Curried Chickpea Stew (page 77)
MONDAY	*Leftover* Blueberry-Nut Oatmeal	*Leftover* Curried Chickpea Stew	*Leftover* Asian-Inspired Turkey Loaf Baked sweet potato (1) (page 71, see tip) *Leftover* Grain-Free Roll (1)
TUESDAY	Fiber Powerhouse Blu-Bana Smoothie (page 42)	*Leftover* Asian-Inspired Turkey Loaf Baked sweet potato (1) (page 71, see tip)	Chicken-Apple Sausage and Pumpkin Soup (page 54) *Leftover* Grain-Free Roll (1)
WEDNESDAY	*Leftover* Fiber Powerhouse Blu-Bana Smoothie	*Leftover* Chicken-Apple Sausage and Pumpkin Soup	*Leftover* Curried Chickpea Stew
THURSDAY	Pumpkin Spice Muffins (2) (page 39)	*Leftover* Chicken-Apple Sausage and Pumpkin Soup *Leftover* Grain-Free Roll (1)	Spaghetti Squash with Clam Sauce (page 74)
FRIDAY	*Leftover* Pumpkin Spice Muffins (2)	*Leftover* Spaghetti Squash with Clam Sauce	Thai-Inspired Flatbreads (page 97)
SATURDAY	*Leftover* Pumpkin Spice Muffins (2)	*Leftover* Thai-Inspired Flatbreads	*Leftover* Spaghetti Squash with Clam Sauce

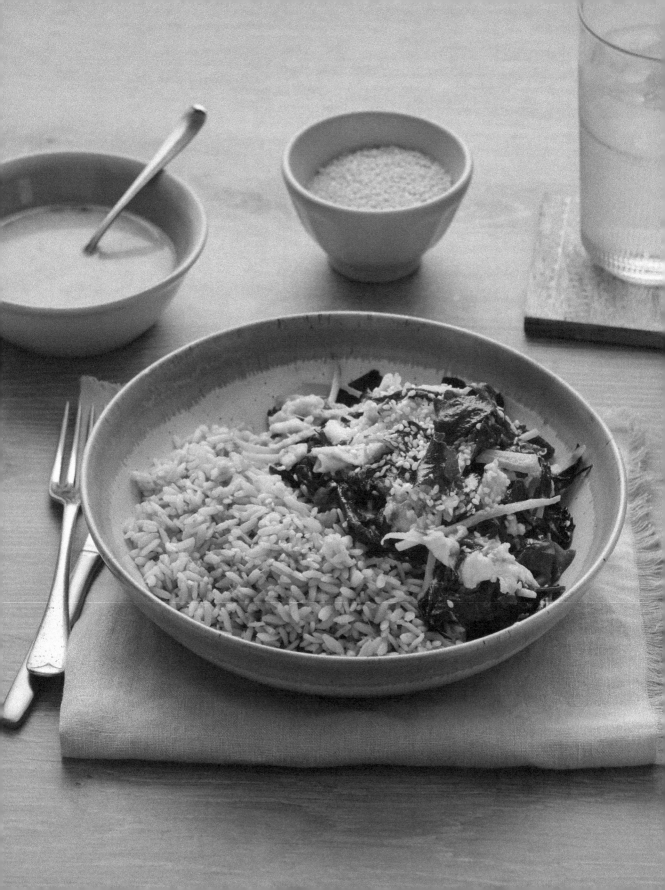

Chapter 2

BREAKFAST AND BEVERAGES

TART CHERRY ELECTROLYTE DRINK

Prep time: 5 minutes | **Makes** 3 servings

The coconut water, honey, and salt provide the electrolytes in this drink. The tart cherry juice provides polyphenols, anthocyanins, melatonin, and tryptophan to help fight heart disease, cancer, cognitive decline, and poor sleep.

1½ cups 100 percent tart cherry juice

1 cup raw coconut water

2 tablespoons raw local honey

⅛ teaspoon Himalayan pink salt

1. In a blender, combine the cherry juice, coconut water, honey, and salt and blend on high for about 15 seconds, until the honey dissolves and is thoroughly incorporated.

2. Chill and serve cold. Store in half-pint mason jars or containers with lids for up to 5 days in the refrigerator or freeze for up to 3 months. For a slushy drink, remove it from the freezer 30 to 60 minutes before consuming.

> **TIP:** If tart cherry juice isn't your thing, you can substitute blueberry or another 100 percent berry juice. After the Clear Liquid Phase, you could add a pinch of cinnamon and/or ginger.

Per serving (7 ounces): Calories: 122; Total fat: 0g; Total carbs: 31g; Cholesterol: 0mg; Fiber: 0g; Sugar: 26g; Protein: 1g; Sodium: 101mg

POMEGRANATE ELECTROLYTE DRINK

Prep time: 5 minutes | **Makes** 3 servings

Pomegranates have polyphenols with potential antioxidant, anti-inflammatory, and anticarcinogenic effects and punicic acid that can help combat high blood sugar, high cholesterol, and high blood pressure. This recipe uses Himalayan pink salt for its trace mineral content and flavor. The honey and baking soda also help support electrolyte balance. Be sure to read labels when buying juice to ensure it doesn't contain added sugars or other unallowable ingredients; not many of them are truly 100 percent juice.

3¾ cups filtered water

1½ cups unsweetened pomegranate juice

1½ tablespoons raw local honey

¼ teaspoon baking soda

¼ teaspoon Himalayan pink salt

1. In a 2-quart pitcher or jar, combine the water, pomegranate juice, honey, baking soda, and salt. Stir or shake to blend.

2. Enjoy immediately or store in pint-size mason jars or containers with lids in the refrigerator for up to 5 days.

> **TIP:** Blueberry juice or pomegranate-blueberry juice is also delicious in this recipe. In the Low-Fiber and High-Fiber Phases, you can add 1 to 2 tablespoons of collagen peptides.

Per serving (12 ounces): Calories: 107; Total fat: 0g; Total carbs: 27g; Cholesterol: 0mg; Fiber: 0g; Sugar: 25g; Protein: 0g; Sodium: 140mg

CRAN-APPLE ELECTROLYTE SLUSHIE

Prep time: 5 minutes | **Makes** 4 servings

This drink combines the sweet taste of apples, the crisp and clean taste of cranberries, and a slushy texture for a sensory treat. The apple and cranberry juices provide antioxidants and a healthy dose of vitamin C to support your immune system. Be sure to use clear or filtered apple juice, rather than cloudy apple juice.

2 cups filtered water

1½ cups filtered apple juice

⅔ cup unsweetened cranberry juice

⅓ cup raw local honey

¼ teaspoon Himalayan pink salt

6 cups ice cubes

1. In a blender, combine the water, apple juice, cranberry juice, honey, and salt and blend on high for about 15 seconds, until the honey is dissolved and thoroughly incorporated.

2. Add the ice cubes and blend thoroughly for 15 to 30 seconds, until the texture is slushy.

3. Enjoy immediately or store in pint-size mason jars or containers with lids and freeze for up to 3 months. For a slushy drink, remove it from the freezer 30 to 60 minutes before consuming. If desired, you can blend it again until slushy.

> **TIP:** Once you're past the Clear Liquid Phase, you can add coconut milk or a nut milk to make this creamy, if desired, and/or substitute orange juice for apple juice.

Per serving (16 ounces): Calories: 149; Total fat: 0g; Total carbs: 39g; Cholesterol: 0mg; Fiber: 0g; Sugar: 39g; Protein: 1g; Sodium: 116mg

BERRY SLUSHIE

Prep time: 5 minutes | **Makes** 4 servings

Berries are among the healthiest foods available. They are good for your heart and your skin, are anti-inflammatory, are loaded with antioxidants, and taste great! This slushie is easy, refreshing, and delicious. If your store doesn't carry Very Berry Juice, use any unsweetened berry juice(s).

2 ½ cups **Very Berry Juice (or another unsweetened berry juice)**

1 cup **raw coconut water**

2 tablespoons **raw local honey**

¼ teaspoon **Himalayan pink salt**

¼ teaspoon **baking soda**

3 cups **ice cubes**

1. In a blender, combine the juice, coconut water, honey, salt, and baking soda and blend for about 15 seconds, until the honey is dissolved and thoroughly incorporated.

2. Add the ice cubes and blend for 15 to 30 seconds, until the texture is slushy.

3. Enjoy immediately or store in pint-size mason jars or containers with lids and refrigerate for up to 5 days or freeze for up to 3 months. For a slushy drink, remove it from the freezer 30 to 60 minutes before consuming.

TIP: In the Low-Fiber Phase, you can use coconut milk instead of water, and in the High-Fiber Phase, you can add some whole berries, if desired.

Per serving (16 ounces): Calories: 95; Total fat: 0g; Total carbs: 24g; Cholesterol: 0mg; Fiber: 0g; Sugar: 24g; Protein: 0g; Sodium: 237mg

BANANA MUFFINS

Prep time: 15 minutes | **Cook time:** 15 minutes | **Makes** 12 muffins

Who doesn't like the smell of sweet banana bread baking? This variation, made into muffins, bakes in a quarter of the time it takes to bake a loaf. As an easy grab-and-go breakfast or snack, muffins are great for meal prepping.

¼ cup coconut oil, plus more for greasing

3 medium extra-ripe bananas

2 large eggs

¼ cup raw local honey

2 cups Low-Fiber Flour Blend (page 119)

1 teaspoon ground cinnamon

1 teaspoon baking powder

½ teaspoon baking soda

⅛ teaspoon sea salt

1. Preheat the oven to 375°F. Grease 12 cups of a muffin tin with coconut oil or line with cupcake liners and set aside.

2. In a blender, combine the bananas, eggs, honey, and oil and blend on high for about 30 seconds, until the oil is thoroughly incorporated. Add the flour blend, cinnamon, baking powder, baking soda, and salt. Blend for 30 to 45 seconds, until the batter is mixed well.

3. Ladle the batter into the prepared muffin tin, filling each cup about half full. Bake for 15 minutes, or until the tops are nicely browned and a toothpick inserted in the middle comes out clean.

4. Once cooled, serve or store in an airtight bag or container at room temperature for up to 2 days, in the refrigerator for up to 5 days, or in the freezer for up to 3 months.

TIP: If you don't have the Low-Fiber Flour Blend made, you can use 1½ cups of white rice flour, ¼ cup of tapioca starch/flour, ¼ cup of arrowroot starch/flour, and 1 teaspoon of xanthan gum.

Per serving (1 muffin): Calories: 199; Total fat: 6.5g; Total carbs: 33g; Cholesterol: 31mg; Fiber: 1g; Sugar: 9.5g; Protein: 2g; Sodium: 99mg

CREAMY CINNAMON-RICE PORRIDGE

Prep time: 10 minutes | **Cook time:** 15 minutes | **Makes** 4 servings

If you grew up loving Cream of Wheat or Cream of Rice, this is a great alternative. Although easily digestible, boxed Cream of Rice is highly processed with synthetic vitamins that aren't good for some people. You can use your favorite short-grain rice in the Low-Fiber Phase and long-grain or brown rice in the High-Fiber Phase, cooked according to the package directions. If desired, top with allowable fruit or berries.

1⅓ cups Arborio rice or other short-grain rice

2 tablespoons collagen peptides

3⅓ cups unsweetened almond milk, plus more if necessary

½ teaspoon sea salt

2 teaspoons raw local honey (optional)

¼ teaspoon ground cinnamon (optional)

1. In a blender or coffee grinder, grind the rice until the pieces are about one-third the original size, or chunkier if you prefer. Don't grind too much, or you'll end up with flour and lumpy porridge. Manually stir in the collagen.

2. In a medium saucepan, bring the milk to a slow boil over medium heat. Add the salt and the rice mixture to the milk gradually, while stirring.

3. Cover and simmer for up to 15 minutes, stirring occasionally to prevent sticking, until thickened. Add water or more milk, if necessary. Turn off the heat, add the honey (if using) and cinnamon (if using), and stir to thoroughly incorporate.

4. Refrigerate the porridge in an airtight container for up to 4 days.

> **TIP:** It won't be as creamy, but you can use water instead of almond milk. In the High-Fiber Phase, use macadamia nut milk or coconut milk for extra creaminess.

Per serving: Calories: 286; Total fat: 3g; Total carbs: 52g; Cholesterol: 0mg; Fiber: 2.5g; Sugar: 0g; Protein: 13g; Sodium: 469mg

SIMPLE BANANA PANCAKES

Prep time: 5 minutes | **Cook time:** 10 minutes | **Makes** 2 servings

These pancakes are quick and easy to whip up for breakfast or when you want breakfast for dinner. They can also be made in advance and refrigerated for up to 5 days or frozen for up to 3 months for pancakes on demand. Putting parchment paper between the pancakes keeps them from sticking together and allows you to take out only the number you want. They reheat nicely in the toaster or microwave. Serve topped with ghee or butter, pure maple syrup, and/or fresh berries, if desired.

1 cup Low-Fiber Flour Blend (page 119)

1 large ripe banana

½ cup unsweetened almond milk

1 large egg

1 teaspoon pure vanilla extract

½ teaspoon ground cinnamon

1 tablespoon coconut oil

1. In a blender, combine the flour blend, banana, milk, egg, vanilla, and cinnamon. Blend on high for about 30 seconds, or until smooth and creamy.

2. In a large nonstick skillet, heat the coconut oil over medium heat or on a griddle at 325°F. When a drop of water dropped on the cooking surface dances and sizzles, pour the batter onto the surface to form 6 pancakes. You'll have to do this in batches if you're using a skillet.

3. Cook for 3 to 4 minutes, until the edges have bubbles, then gently flip. Cook for another 3 to 4 minutes, until both sides are brown and the centers aren't gooey.

4. Serve hot.

> **TIP:** In a pinch, you can use 1 cup of white rice flour plus 2 teaspoons of baking powder instead of the flour blend.

Per serving (3 [4-inch] pancakes): Calories: 412; Total fat: 10g; Total carbs: 71g; Cholesterol: 93mg; Fiber: 2.5g; Sugar: 7.5g; Protein: 6g; Sodium: 113mg

BROCCOLI, TOMATO, AND QUINOA FRITTATA

Prep time: 15 minutes | **Cook time:** 25 minutes | **Makes** 6 servings

This breakfast comes together quickly when using precooked quinoa and frozen broccoli. Batch-cooking grains on Sunday makes for quick weekday meals. Use broth instead of water for extra nutrition and flavor.

10 ounces frozen chopped broccoli

1 tablespoon coconut oil

6 large eggs

1½ cups cooked quinoa

3 medium Roma tomatoes, seeded and chopped

3 large scallions, green parts only, chopped

1 large ripe avocado, pitted, peeled, and diced

½ teaspoon sea salt

Pinch ground black pepper

1. Rinse the broccoli and put it in a strainer to drain for about 30 minutes, or microwave it for about 2 minutes and drain any excess liquid.

2. Meanwhile, preheat the oven to 400°F. Grease a 9½- to 10-inch pie plate with the coconut oil and set aside.

3. In a large bowl, beat the eggs. Fold in the quinoa, broccoli, tomatoes, scallions, avocado, salt, and pepper. Pour the egg mixture into the prepared pie plate.

4. Bake for 20 to 25 minutes, or until the egg is set. Allow to cool in the pan for 5 to 10 minutes before cutting into 6 wedges and serving.

5. Serve or store in airtight containers in the refrigerator for up to 5 days or in the freezer up to 3 months.

TIP: To cook quinoa, rinse it, then stir and toast it in the pan before adding twice as much liquid as quinoa. Bring to a boil and then simmer, covered, until the quinoa is tender and looks like it has popped open, about 15 minutes.

Per serving (1 wedge): Calories: 223; Total fat: 12g; Total carbs: 17g; Cholesterol: 186mg; Fiber: 5g; Sugar: 3g; Protein: 10g; Sodium: 288mg

WAKAME BOWL

Prep time: 15 minutes | **Cook time:** 10 minutes | **Makes** 6 servings

After enjoying a wakame bowl at a former cafe in Moab, Utah, and butchering the pronunciation, I had to recreate it. *Wakame* (pronounced wah-KAH-meh) is an edible seaweed that even in small amounts is mineral rich and helps combat heart disease, cancer, and diabetes. Precooked rice makes for quick prep. Buy it precooked or cook and refrigerate what you need for the next week.

3 ounces dried wakame

2 large garlic cloves

1 (1-inch) piece ginger, peeled

3 tablespoons reduced-sodium tamari

3 tablespoons raw local honey

4 teaspoons sesame oil

1 tablespoon rice vinegar

6 tablespoons olive oil, divided

6 scallions, green parts only, thinly sliced

3 small carrots, shredded

9 large eggs, beaten

6 cups cooked brown rice

Black and/or white sesame seeds, for garnish (optional)

1. In a small bowl, soak the wakame in hot water while you prepare the sauce and eggs.

2. In a food processor or blender, combine the garlic, ginger, tamari, honey, sesame oil, and vinegar and process until the ginger and garlic are pureed. With the food processor or blender running, slowly stream in 5 tablespoons of olive oil. Blend until the sauce looks a little creamy. Set aside.

3. In a medium skillet, heat the remaining 1 tablespoon of olive oil over medium-high heat until hot but not smoking. Add the scallions and carrots and sauté for 3 to 4 minutes, or until the scallions are fragrant.

4. Reduce the heat to medium-low. Add the eggs and let them cook until you see the bottom start to set. Using a silicon spatula, gently scrape the bottom and sides of the pan and turn the eggs for 3 to 5 minutes, just until they are set. Turn the heat off.

5. Drain any excess liquid from the wakame. Add the wakame to the eggs and stir gently. Serve the eggs over the rice in bowls. Drizzle with the sauce and garnish with sesame seeds (if using).

TIP: Feel free to use liquid egg whites or a combination of whole eggs and egg whites. I've included a source for wakame in the Resources section (see page 130) if you can't find it. Wakame has a unique flavor, but you can use dulse or omit it.

Per serving: Calories: 559; Total fat: 26g; Total carbs: 65g; Cholesterol: 279mg; Fiber: 5g; Sugar: 11g; Protein: 16g; Sodium: 981mg

PEACH SMOOTHIE

Prep time: 5 minutes | **Makes** 2 servings

This smoothie can be made with coconut water for electrolytes or a nut milk for extra creaminess. Be sure to buy peaches packed in juice rather than syrup. For the early Low-Fiber Phase, I recommend using coconut water. The avocado and ice will provide some healthy fat and great texture.

1 cup coconut water or unsweetened almond milk

1 (15-ounce) can juice-packed sliced peaches

½ medium avocado, pitted and peeled

2 tablespoons collagen peptides

1 cup ice cubes

1. In a blender, combine the coconut water, peaches, avocado, and collagen. Process on high speed for about 15 seconds until smooth. Add the ice and blend until it reaches your desired consistency.

2. Enjoy immediately or store in jars or containers with lids in the refrigerator for up to 2 days.

TIP: To save a partial avocado, retain the pit and peel. Sprinkle lemon juice on the remaining avocado. Put the peeled halves and pit back together, wrap tightly with plastic wrap, and refrigerate.

Per serving (2 cups): Calories: 197; Total fat: 5.5g; Total carbs: 33g; Cholesterol: 0mg; Fiber: 5g; Sugar: 27g; Protein: 8g; Sodium: 63mg

PUMPKIN SPICE MUFFINS

Prep time: 15 minutes | **Cook time:** 20 minutes | **Makes** 12 muffins

Fall is pumpkin spice season, but pumpkin is available year-round, so why limit yourself? These quick muffins are great for breakfast, brunch, dessert, or a snack. The raisins and pecans help get these to 5.5 grams of fiber but can be optional if you're not yet ready to add them in.

3 tablespoons coconut oil, melted, plus more for greasing the pan

6 large eggs

¾ cup pumpkin puree

6 tablespoons raw local honey

1½ teaspoons pure vanilla extract

6 tablespoons arrowroot starch/ flour

6 tablespoons coconut flour

1½ teaspoons baking soda

¾ teaspoon pumpkin pie spice

¼ teaspoon sea salt

½ cup raisins

½ cup chopped pecans

1. Preheat the oven to 375°F. Grease 12 cups of a muffin tin with coconut oil and set aside.

2. In a large bowl, beat the eggs. Whisk in the pumpkin puree, honey, vanilla, and melted coconut oil until the honey is thoroughly incorporated.

3. Add the arrowroot, coconut flour, baking soda, pumpkin pie spice, and salt. Stir the mixture until all the dry ingredients are moistened. Fold in the raisins and pecans.

4. Ladle the batter into the prepared muffin tin, filling each cup about completely full. The batter will be runny, but the coconut flour and raisins will absorb the liquid.

5. Bake for 20 minutes, or until a toothpick inserted in the center comes out clean.

6. Once cooled, serve or store in an airtight bag or container at room temperature for up to 2 days, in the refrigerator for up to 5 days, or in the freezer up to 3 months.

TIP: You can make bread instead of muffins using a 9 x 5-inch loaf pan. Bake for 1 hour, or until a toothpick inserted in the center comes out clean.

Per serving (2 muffins): Calories: 389; Total fat: 20g; Total carbs: 44g; Cholesterol: 186mg; Fiber: 5.5g; Sugar: 28g; Protein: 9g; Sodium: 501mg

CARROT CAKE SMOOTHIE

Prep time: 10 minutes | **Cook time:** 5 minutes | **Makes** 2 servings

This smoothie gets extra sweetness from the frozen ripe banana and richness from the coconut milk. When my bananas start to turn black, I peel them and freeze them. Then, whenever I want to make a smoothie or banana bread, I have ripe bananas on hand.

2 medium carrots, shredded

1 cup full-fat coconut milk

2 medium frozen ripe bananas

¼ cup collagen peptides

2 teaspoons raw local honey, plus more if needed

1 teaspoon pure vanilla extract

¼ teaspoon ground cinnamon

¼ teaspoon ground nutmeg

2 cups ice cubes

1. In a large pot that fits a steamer basket or insert, bring 1 inch of water to a boil. Put the carrots into the steamer basket and place it in the pot. Cover and cook for 5 minutes, until fork-tender.

2. In a blender, combine the steamed carrots with the coconut milk, bananas, collagen, honey, vanilla, cinnamon, and nutmeg. Blend on high for about 15 seconds, or until smooth. Taste and adjust the honey, if desired. Add the ice cubes and blend again for 15 to 30 seconds to your desired consistency.

3. Serve immediately or store in mason jars or containers with lids in the refrigerator for up to 2 days.

TIP: For a delicious higher-fiber version, use raw carrot and add ¼ cup of gluten-free rolled oats, ⅓ cup of frozen pineapple chunks, and 2 tablespoons of ground flaxseed.

Per serving (18 ounces): Calories: 429; Total fat: 25g; Total carbs: 42g; Cholesterol: 0mg; Fiber: 6g; Sugar: 23g; Protein: 16g; Sodium: 100mg

SWEET POTATO, AVOCADO, AND EGG TOAST

Prep time: 10 minutes | **Cook time:** 30 minutes | **Makes** 4 servings

Sweet potato slices are the new healthy toast. Topped with avocado and egg, this makes a delicious and nutritious breakfast. I like poached eggs on mine, but you can bake, boil, or scramble your eggs if you prefer. Sweet potato toast is also delicious topped with bean or artichoke dip.

2 medium sweet potatoes, sliced lengthwise into 8 (½-inch-thick) planks

1 tablespoon olive oil

½ teaspoon sea salt

2 medium avocados, pitted, peeled, and mashed

4 large eggs, cooked as desired

1. Preheat the oven to 400°F. Line a baking sheet with parchment paper and set aside.

2. In a large bowl, toss the sweet potatoes with the oil and season with the salt. Arrange the slices in a single layer on the baking sheet and roast for about 30 minutes, turning once after 15 minutes, until the sweet potatoes are tender and begin to caramelize.

3. Transfer them to a wire rack and let them cool completely.

4. To serve, on each sweet potato slice, spread the mashed avocado and top with cooked egg. Plain sweet potato toast slices can be refrigerated in an airtight container for up to 5 days. To reheat, warm the slices in a toaster oven until crisp, about 2 minutes, and top them with avocado and egg.

TIP: If you'll be storing or meal prepping these, be sure to use sweet potatoes and not yams, because yams get mushy.

Per serving (2 slices): Calories: 271; Total fat: 19g; Total carbs: 19g; Cholesterol: 186mg; Fiber: 6.5g; Sugar: 3g; Protein: 9g; Sodium: 403mg

FIBER POWERHOUSE BLU-BANA SMOOTHIE

Prep time: 5 minutes | **Makes** 3 servings

This is like dessert for breakfast. If you let it sit or refrigerate it, the flax and chia seeds will thicken up like yummy pudding. Blueberries are not only a delicious brain food but also protect against heart disease, improve bone health, encourage blood circulation, and help control blood sugar levels.

1¼ teaspoons pumpkin seeds

1¼ teaspoons chia seeds

1¼ teaspoons psyllium husk powder

1½ cups frozen blueberries

1 large frozen banana

1 cup full-fat coconut milk

2 tablespoons collagen peptides

2 tablespoons pure creamy almond butter

1¼ teaspoons ground flaxseed

1 to 2 teaspoons raw local honey (optional)

1 cup filtered water or ice, or to desired consistency

1. In a high-speed blender, combine the pumpkin seeds, chia seeds, and psyllium. Blend on high for about 15 seconds until powdery. Add the blueberries, banana, coconut milk, collagen, almond butter, flaxseed, and honey (if using). Blend until smooth, about 2 minutes. Add water or ice, if needed, and blend again to reach your desired consistency.

2. Enjoy immediately or store in pint-size jars or containers with lids in the refrigerator for up to 2 days.

TIP: Always store flaxseed in the freezer. You can substitute any berry or combination of berries for the blueberries.

Per serving: Calories: 311; Total fat: 23g; Total carbs: 21g; Cholesterol: 0mg; Fiber: 7g; Sugar: 9.5g; Protein: 9g; Sodium: 32mg

BLUEBERRY-NUT OATMEAL

Prep time: 5 minutes | **Cook time:** 10 minutes | **Makes** 2 servings

This sweet, earthy oatmeal is comforting and delicious. The healthy dose of fiber will keep you satisfied and support your microbiome and digestion. This dish is also heart-healthy with antioxidants and healthy fats. Since avoiding nuts is no longer advised after recovery, I've included almond butter and almonds. Omit them, of course, if nuts are a trigger food for you.

1½ cups filtered water

¼ teaspoon sea salt

1 cup gluten-free rolled oats

2 tablespoons raw local honey, plus more for drizzling

2 tablespoons pure creamy almond butter

1 teaspoon ground cinnamon

½ cup unsweetened almond milk

¾ cup blueberries

1½ tablespoons chopped raw or dry-roasted almonds

1½ tablespoons shredded unsweetened coconut

2 teaspoons ground flaxseed

1. In a medium saucepan over high heat, bring the water and salt to a boil. Add the oats and stir. Reduce the heat to low and simmer, stirring occasionally, for 10 minutes, or until thickened. (Cooking for 10 to 15 minutes longer will result in creamier oats, but be careful not to scorch the bottom.)

2. Remove the pan from the heat. Stir in the honey, almond butter, and cinnamon.

3. Serve with the milk and top with blueberries, almonds, coconut, and flaxseed. Drizzle with more honey, if desired. Store the oatmeal without toppings in an airtight container and refrigerate up to 4 days or freeze for up to 3 months.

TIP: I recommend raw nuts that have been soaked or sprouted to reduce the antinutrients and make them more digestible (see Resources, page 130).

Per serving: Calories: 452; Total fat: 18g; Total carbs: 68g; Cholesterol: 0mg; Fiber: 9.5g; Sugar: 34g; Protein: 11g; Sodium: 340mg

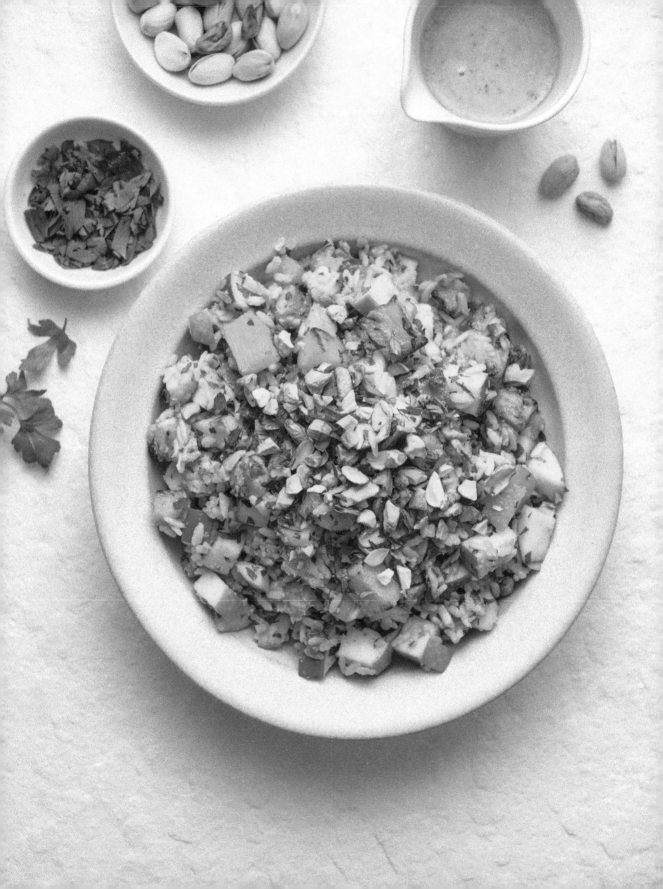

Chapter 3

SOUPS AND SALADS

LOW-FODMAP VEGETABLE BROTH

Prep time: 15 minutes | **Cook time:** 1 hour 20 minutes | **Makes** 8 cups

Strain this tasty broth through cheesecloth for the Clear Liquid Phase and use it as a base for your favorite soup, noodles, or dumplings once you've healed. The green parts of the leeks and oyster mushrooms keep this low-FODMAP (use 3 leeks if you don't have many green parts from 2). Since you'll be discarding or composting the veggies, don't worry about peeling or chopping them beautifully or even removing the parsley stems.

12 cups filtered water

8 ounces oyster mushrooms, roughly chopped

4 medium carrots, cut into 1-inch pieces

2 large leeks, green parts only, cleaned and cut into ½-inch strips

2 small celeriac, peeled and cut into 1-inch cubes

½ bunch fresh flat-leaf parsley, cut into thirds

4 thyme sprigs

2 bay leaves

1 teaspoon sea salt

1. In a large stockpot or Dutch oven, combine the water, mushrooms, carrots, leeks, celeriac, parsley, thyme, bay leaves, and salt. Bring the contents to a boil over high heat. Cover the pot and reduce the heat as needed to keep it at a low boil for 1 hour.

2. Strain the vegetables through a cheesecloth-lined mesh strainer and store the broth in an airtight container in the refrigerator for up to 4 days or in the freezer up to 6 months.

TIP: To use an Instant Pot, dump everything in and cook on high pressure for 30 minutes. You can buy ready-made vegetable broth that may even be less expensive, but it won't be as tasty or low-FODMAP.

Per serving (1 cup): Calories: 9; Total fat: 0g; Total carbs: 2g; Cholesterol: 0mg; Fiber: 0g; Sugar: 1g; Protein: 0g; Sodium: 316mg

CREAMY LEMON AND RICE SOUP WITH CHICKEN

Prep time: 10 minutes | **Cook time:** 30 minutes | **Makes** 4 servings

This one-pot soup is adapted from a Greek soup called avgolemono. This is a low-fiber dish, but after you've recovered, add red or black pepper and pair it with Grain-Free Rolls (page 124) or salad.

2 tablespoons olive oil

3 medium scallions, green parts only, diced

⅔ cup Arborio rice or other short-grain white rice

½ teaspoon sea salt

4 cups Chicken Bone Broth (page 114)

2 cups unsweetened almond milk

5 ounces Tender Stewed Chicken, shredded (page 117)

4 large eggs

Juice of 1 lemon

1. In a large saucepan, heat the oil over medium heat. Add the scallions and cook for 3 minutes, stirring, until very tender.

2. Increase the heat to medium-high, stir in the rice, and cook for 1 to 2 minutes, until the rice is fragrant. Season with salt.

3. Stir in the broth. Bring to a boil over high heat, then reduce the heat to low. Cover and simmer for 20 minutes. Stir in the milk and chicken.

4. In small bowl, beat the eggs and lemon juice. While stirring constantly, slowly add 1 cup of hot soup to the egg mixture.

5. Turn the heat to low. Slowly stream the egg mixture into the soup. Heat the soup through, but don't boil it.

6. Enjoy immediately or refrigerate for up 4 days or freeze for up to 3 months.

TIP: You can swap a 5-ounce can of chicken with its liquid for the shredded chicken.

Per serving: Calories: 374; Total fat: 15g; Total carbs: 28g; Cholesterol: 220mg; Fiber: 1.5g; Sugar: 1g; Protein: 29g; Sodium: 825mg

CHICKEN-CELERIAC SOUP WITH TARRAGON

Prep time: 10 minutes | **Cook time:** 25 minutes | **Makes** 3 servings

This easy soup is comforting on a cool day. The bittersweet, mild licorice flavor of tarragon pairs beautifully with the celeriac (celery root). It freezes well so it's perfect for meal prepping.

3 cups Chicken Bone Broth (page 114)

2 cups unsweetened almond milk

1 large celeriac, peeled and cut into ½-inch cubes

½ teaspoon sea salt

1 teaspoon dried tarragon

2 tablespoons arrowroot starch/flour

3 tablespoons cold filtered water

6 ounces Tender Stewed Chicken, shredded (page 117)

1. In a large saucepan or Dutch oven, bring the broth, milk, celeriac, and salt to a boil over high heat. Cover and reduce the heat as needed to maintain a simmer for 20 minutes. Add the tarragon in the last few minutes.

2. In a small bowl or cup, whisk the arrowroot into the water. Add the mixture to the soup and stir for about 3 minutes, or until it thickens.

3. Once cooked, blend with an immersion blender to create a thick soup, leaving some chunks. If you don't have an immersion blender, carefully transfer all but 1 to 2 cups of the soup from the pan to a food processor or blender. Puree it and then add the puree back to the pot; stir in the chicken and heat through.

4. Serve immediately or store in an airtight container in the refrigerator for up to 4 days or in the freezer for up to 3 months.

TIP: To add more fiber, consider substituting 1 cup of cooked white beans for the chicken. For variety, use 1 tablespoon of fresh chopped tarragon, rosemary, or parsley instead of the dried tarragon.

Per serving: Calories: 229; Total fat: 6g; Total carbs: 15g; Cholesterol: 51mg; Fiber: 2g; Sugar: 2g; Protein: 27g; Sodium: 1,013mg

TUNA SALAD WITH AVOCADO

Prep time: 10 minutes | **Makes** 3 servings

This dish is a twist on classic tuna salad. The avocado adds flavor, creamy texture, and healthy fat, along with nearly 3 grams of fiber. It is a great go-to recipe for a quick, easy lunch or dinner.

3 tablespoons avocado oil mayonnaise

¼ teaspoon sea salt

Pinch dried basil

7½ ounces water-packed albacore chunk tuna, drained

¾ small avocado, pitted, peeled, and diced

1. In a medium bowl, whisk together the mayonnaise, salt, and basil. Gently fold in the tuna.

2. Add the avocado just before serving so it doesn't turn brown. For the Low-Fiber Phase, serve this alone or on white bread. For the High-Fiber Phase, serve it on a bed of salad greens or whole-grain bread.

3. Chill if not serving immediately. Store in an airtight container in the refrigerator for up to 3 days.

TIP: For variety: (1) Sprinkle with paprika and a chiffonade of fresh basil leaves instead of dried; (2) add 8 sliced Castelvetrano or other green olives; or (3) use chicken instead of tuna.

Per serving: Calories: 228; Total fat: 18g; Total carbs: 3g; Cholesterol: 50mg; Fiber: 2.5g; Sugar: 0g; Protein: 16g; Sodium: 487mg

EASY CHICKEN AND RICE NOODLE SOUP

Prep time: 15 minutes | **Cook time:** 20 minutes | **Makes** 4 servings

This soup uses celeriac (celery root) instead of celery, which tastes like celery, is low-FODMAP, and has no strings. You can use ready-made bone broth and any leftover, deli, or canned chicken.

2 tablespoons olive oil

2 medium carrots, peeled and diced into ¼-inch pieces

½ large celeriac (celery root), peeled and diced into ¼-inch pieces

4 cups Chicken Bone Broth (page 114)

4 ounces rice sticks (thin rice noodles/rice vermicelli)

10 ounces Tender Stewed Chicken, shredded (page 117)

1 teaspoon sea salt

1. In a large stockpot or Dutch oven, heat the oil over medium-high heat. Add the carrots and celeriac. Sauté for 5 minutes.

2. Add the broth. Bring the mixture to a boil over high heat. Reduce the heat as needed to maintain a low boil for about 10 minutes, or until the vegetables are soft enough to mash with a fork.

3. Meanwhile, in a large saucepan, bring about 2 inches of water to a boil. Add the rice sticks and cook for 3 minutes, or until the noodles are just softening. Stir and watch carefully to avoid overcooking. Drain.

4. Add the noodles and the chicken to the broth. Season with salt. Reduce the heat to low and cook for about 2 minutes to warm the chicken.

5. Serve immediately or divide into individual airtight containers and store in the refrigerator for 5 days or freeze for up to 3 months.

> **TIP:** After recovery, don't peel the carrots, use a high-fiber noodle, and if tolerated, add garlic and ground black pepper.

Per serving: Calories: 329; Total fat: 12g; Total carbs: 33g; Cholesterol: 58mg; Fiber: 2.5g; Sugar: 3g; Protein: 22g; Sodium: 237mg

TURKEY ALBONDIGAS SOUP

Prep time: 15 minutes | **Cook time:** 30 minutes | **Makes** 4 servings

Albondigas means "meatballs." The zucchini in this meatball soup adds texture and thickness, is anti-inflammatory, benefits digestive health, and provides electrolytes. For the High-Fiber Phase, skip peeling the vegetables and serve topped with chopped cilantro, avocado, and a squeeze of lime.

¾ cup cooked Arborio rice

1 pound ground turkey

2 medium scallions, green parts only, thinly sliced

½ teaspoon sea salt

¼ teaspoon dried Mexican oregano

8 cups Chicken Bone Broth (page 114)

¾ cup tomato juice

2 large carrots, peeled and cubed

2 small zucchini, peeled and sliced horizontally (⅜ inch thick)

1 large russet potato, peeled and cubed

1. In a medium bowl, thoroughly mix the turkey, rice, scallions, salt, and oregano and set aside.

2. In a medium stockpot, boil the chicken broth over medium-high heat.

3. Using a meat baller or by hand, shape the meat-rice mixture into 1-inch balls and drop them into the boiling broth. Cook for 5 minutes.

4. Add the tomato juice, carrots, zucchini, and potato to the stockpot. Boil for 25 minutes, or until the vegetables are soft and the meatballs reach an internal temperature of 165°F or are no longer pink in the center.

5. Serve promptly, or store in an airtight container in the refrigerator for up to 3 days or in the freezer for up to 3 months.

TIP: To save time, use an Instant Pot or rice cooker to batch-cook rice or buy precooked rice. I like to cook my rice in chicken broth.

Per serving: Calories: 408; Total fat: 9g; Total carbs: 36g; Cholesterol: 88mg; Fiber: 4g; Sugar: 6g; Protein: 44g; Sodium: 1,000mg

HERB AND FLAKED FISH SOUP

Prep time: 15 minutes, plus 8 hours to soak | **Cook time:** 10 minutes
Makes 4 servings

This bright-green soup has amazing depth of flavor and a velvety texture. The cashews add creaminess and contribute to the fiber content along with the peas and spinach. The lime gives it just the right amount of tang to complement the fish.

2 cod fillets
   (5 to 6 ounces each)

1 tablespoon ground
   turmeric

½ teaspoon sea salt,
   divided

¼ teaspoon ground
   black pepper, divided

16 ounces frozen peas

3 cups Chicken Bone
   Broth, divided
   (page 114)

5 ounces frozen spinach

¼ cup raw cashews,
   soaked overnight
   and drained

1 handful fresh cilantro,
   plus 2 tablespoons for
   garnish

1 handful fresh flat-leaf
   parsley, large stems
   removed

3 large scallions, green
   parts only, roughly
   chopped

3 medium limes, 1 juiced
   and 2 cut into wedges

1. Preheat the oven to 350°F. Line a baking sheet with parchment paper and set aside.

2. Pat the fish dry. Sprinkle them with the turmeric, ¼ teaspoon of the salt, and ⅛ teaspoon of the pepper and place them on the lined baking sheet. Bake for 5 minutes and flip the fillets over. Bake for another 5 minutes, or until the fish reaches 145°F and flakes easily with a fork. Remove the fish from the oven and roughly flake it with a fork.

3. While the fish is cooking, in a large saucepan, combine the peas and 2½ cups of broth and bring to a boil over medium-high heat. Cook for 5 minutes. Add the spinach; allow it to thaw and heat through.

4. In a blender set on high speed, blend the cashews with the remaining ½ cup of chicken broth for 30 to 60 seconds until creamy. Add the cilantro, parsley, and scallions and blend for about 30 seconds until smooth.

5. Transfer the saucepan contents to the blender. Add the lime juice and blend until smooth. Season with the remaining ¼ teaspoon of salt and ⅛ teaspoon of pepper.

6. To serve, top the soup with flaked fish and garnish with lime wedges and cilantro. Store the soup, fish, and toppings separately. Refrigerate the soup in an airtight container for up to 5 days and the fish for up to 3 days, or freeze for up to 2 months.

TIP: Great substitutions include chives for the scallions, basil or oregano for the cilantro, and haddock, pollack, black cod, striped bass, hake, mahi-mahi, or grouper for the cod.

Per serving: Calories: 238; Total fat: 4g; Total carbs: 20g; Cholesterol: 40mg; Fiber: 6.5g; Sugar: 6g; Protein: 30g; Sodium: 672mg

CHICKEN-APPLE SAUSAGE AND PUMPKIN SOUP

Prep time: 10 minutes | **Cook time:** 30 minutes | **Makes** 4 servings

The combination of apples, smoked sausage, and mustard gives this soup a bit of Bavarian-like flair with a rich base. The quinoa and pumpkin are anti-inflammatory and contribute fiber and antioxidants. This soup is easy to make and great for meal prepping.

1 tablespoon olive oil

12 ounces chicken and apple sausages, cut into bite-size pieces

1 small onion, chopped

1 teaspoon rubbed sage

1 cup quinoa, rinsed

4 cups Chicken Bone Broth (page 114)

1 (15-ounce) can pumpkin puree

2 tablespoons pure maple syrup

1 tablespoon raw apple cider vinegar

1 tablespoon dry mustard

⅛ teaspoon ground black pepper

1. In 4-quart pot or Dutch oven, heat the oil over medium heat and cook the sausages, onion, and sage for 3 minutes, stirring often. Add the quinoa and broth. Bring to a boil. Reduce the heat to low and cover. Simmer for 15 to 20 minutes, or until the quinoa is tender and looks like it has popped open.

2. Add the pumpkin puree, maple syrup, vinegar, and mustard. Cook for 2 to 3 minutes to heat through. Season with the pepper.

3. Enjoy immediately or store in an airtight container in the refrigerator for up to 5 days or in the freezer for up to 3 months.

TIP: Be sure to read the sausage ingredients to avoid dairy, corn syrup, dextrose, MSG, and nitrites. I use Aidells organic all-natural chicken sausages, which is widely available.

Per serving: Calories: 495; Total fat: 20g; Total carbs: 49g; Cholesterol: 67mg; Fiber: 6g; Sugar: 15g; Protein: 29g; Sodium: 1,100mg

SWEET POTATO-CHICKPEA SALAD

Prep time: 10 minutes, plus 20 minutes to cool | **Cook time:** 25 minutes
Makes 6 servings

This brightly colored salad is rich in polyphenols and fiber. The sweet potatoes, red bell pepper, and orange juice add a delicious sweetness complimented by the warm, spicy cumin and buttery flavor of pine nuts.

2 pounds sweet potatoes, peeled and cut into ½- to ¾-inch cubes

2 large red bell peppers, cut into ½-inch square pieces

¼ cup, plus 2 tablespoons olive oil, divided

½ teaspoon sea salt

1 (15-ounce) can chickpeas, drained and rinsed

⅓ cup chopped fresh flat-leaf parsley

1 tablespoon champagne vinegar

1 tablespoon orange juice

¼ teaspoon ground cumin

⅓ cup lightly toasted pine nuts

1. Preheat the oven to 400°F. Line 2 baking sheets with parchment paper.

2. Put the sweet potatoes and bell peppers on separate prepared baking sheets. Drizzle each with 1 tablespoon of the olive oil and sprinkle with the salt. Toss to coat all the pieces. Spread the veggies out in a single layer. Bake for about 25 minutes, stirring halfway through, until the peppers are slightly charred and the sweet potato cubes are fork-tender. Transfer the baking sheet(s) to cooling racks for about 20 minutes.

3. In a large bowl, combine the sweet potatoes, bell peppers, chickpeas, and parsley.

4. In a small bowl, whisk together the remaining ¼ cup of oil, the vinegar, orange juice, and cumin.

5. Pour the vinegar mixture into the large bowl and toss to combine. Serve immediately garnished with pine nuts or refrigerate in an airtight container for up 5 days.

TIP: Combining sweet potatoes with yams and/or purple sweet potatoes will add even more color to this beautiful salad.

Per serving: Calories: 335; Total fat: 20g; Total carbs: 35g; Cholesterol: 0mg; Fiber: 7g; Sugar: 8.5g; Protein: 6g; Sodium: 339mg

ROOT VEGGIE SLAW

Prep time: 15 minutes | **Cook time:** 5 minutes | **Makes** 8 servings

Different-colored root vegetables provide healthy polyphenols and fiber. The earthy tastes of rainbow carrots, beets, and parsnips are complemented by the cilantro and light vinaigrette dressing. To build your own salad, vary the root vegetables, selecting from celeriac, daikon radish, fennel, turnips, red radish, or rutabagas, and swap the cilantro for your favorite herb.

½ cup chopped walnuts

1 large beet, coarsely shredded

2 large parsnips, coarsely shredded

2 large rainbow carrots, coarsely shredded

½ bunch fresh cilantro

⅓ cup Garlic Oil (page 115) or olive oil

2½ tablespoons freshly squeezed lemon juice

½ teaspoon sea salt

⅛ teaspoon ground black pepper

2 avocados, pitted, peeled, and cubed

1. In a large, dry skillet, toast the walnuts over medium-high heat. Watch them constantly and stir frequently for about 5 minutes, or until the walnuts start to brown and smell toasted. Transfer the walnuts to a plate to cool.

2. In a large bowl, combine the beet, parsnips, carrots, and cilantro.

3. In a separate small bowl, whisk the oil, lemon juice, salt, and pepper. Pour the oil mixture over the veggies and toss to combine.

4. Toss the avocados in when you're ready to serve and garnish with the walnuts. Refrigerate leftovers in an airtight container for 2 to 3 days.

TIP: A food processor with a grating blade isn't necessary but would make shredding the vegetables faster and easier.

Per serving: Calories: 222; Total fat: 12g; Total carbs: 27g; Cholesterol: 5mg; Fiber: 7.5g; Sugar: 5g; Protein: 4g; Sodium: 193mg

WINTER APPLE-SQUASH SALAD

Prep time: 15 minutes | **Cook time:** 30 minutes | **Makes** 4 servings

This is a beautifully colorful dish, which means it has lots of healthy polyphenols. Nutty brown rice; chewy, sweet dates; and crunchy apples contribute to the flavor complexity in this delicious salad.

2 cups cooked
long-grain brown rice

½ cup pitted dates,
soaked, then finely
chopped

2 cups butternut
squash cubes

⅓ cup, plus
2 tablespoons olive oil,
divided

½ cup pistachios,
divided

¼ cup champagne
vinegar

2 teaspoons ground
cardamom

1 teaspoon grated
orange zest

2 cups chopped apples
(½-inch pieces)

1 handful fresh flat-leaf
parsley, stemmed and
chopped

1. Preheat the oven to 400°F. Line a baking sheet with parchment paper and set aside.

2. Put the squash on the baking sheet and drizzle with 2 tablespoons of the oil. Toss to evenly coat the squash. Roast the squash for 25 to 30 minutes, turning once, until tender.

3. Chop and set aside 3 tablespoons of the pistachios.

4. In a blender, combine the remaining ⅓ cup of pistachios, the remaining ⅓ cup of olive oil, the vinegar, cardamom, and orange zest and process until the pistachios are finely chopped.

5. In a large bowl, combine the rice, dates, squash, apples, and parsley. Pour the dressing on top. Toss to coat. Garnish with the reserved pistachios before serving. Refrigerate leftovers in an airtight container for up to 5 days.

TIP: If you can only find frozen squash, cook it straight from the freezer at 450°F for 25 minutes.

Per serving: Calories: 556; Total fat: 33g; Total carbs: 61g; Cholesterol: 0mg; Fiber: 7.5g; Sugar: 22g; Protein: 8g; Sodium: 11mg

MACARONI-SHRIMP SALAD

Prep time: 10 minutes | **Cook time:** 15 minutes | **Makes** 4 servings

This is a remake of my mother's classic macaroni salad. Using lentil pasta bumps up the fiber count, and using an avocado oil mayonnaise provides healthier fats. The slivered, toasted almonds were my own addition to texture and fiber.

9 ounces lentil elbow pasta or another small shape

8 ounces cooked baby shrimp

1⅓ cups frozen peas

1 (4-ounce) jar diced pimentos

3 large scallions, green parts only, sliced

½ cup chopped fresh flat-leaf parsley

½ cup avocado oil mayonnaise

1 tablespoon freshly squeezed lemon juice

½ teaspoon sea salt

¼ cup slivered almonds, toasted

1. Cook the pasta according to the package directions. Drain the pasta and rinse it with cold water. Set aside.

2. Meanwhile, in a large bowl, combine the shrimp, peas, pimentos, scallions, and parsley.

3. In a small bowl, whisk together the mayonnaise, lemon juice, and salt.

4. Toss the pasta with the ingredients in the large bowl. Pour in the mayonnaise mixture and toss to coat the salad ingredients. Garnish with the almonds.

5. Enjoy immediately or store in an airtight container in the refrigerator for up 3 days.

TIP: Most stores have lentil, pea, or chickpea pasta options now, or you can order them online (see Resources, page 130). These options are gluten-free and higher in fiber than most other pasta.

Per serving: Calories: 631; Total fat: 35g; Total carbs: 53g; Cholesterol: 114mg; Fiber: 8.5g; Sugar: 3.5g; Protein: 26g; Sodium: 836mg

FAVA BEAN SOUP

Prep time: 15 minutes | **Cook time:** 10 minutes | **Makes** 4 servings

My friend Justin Soltani taught me how to make this fast, easy, Persian-inspired fava bean soup. Fava beans have a delicious nutty taste and buttery texture. The garlic, cumin, and lemon juice make the fava beans taste fabulous!

2 tablespoons olive oil

4 large garlic cloves, minced

2 (15-ounce) cans fava beans, drained and rinsed

1 cup vegetable broth

½ teaspoon ground cumin

½ teaspoon sea salt

⅛ teaspoon ground black pepper

Juice of 1 large lemon

1 large tomato, seeded and diced, divided

1 handful fresh flat-leaf parsley, stemmed and chopped

1. In a large skillet, heat the olive oil over medium-high heat until hot but not smoking. Add the garlic and sauté for about 30 seconds until fragrant.

2. Add the fava beans, vegetable broth, cumin, salt, and pepper. Cook for about 10 minutes to allow the flavors to blend. Drizzle the mixture with lemon juice as you mash the beans with a potato masher or fork, tasting as you go so you can adjust the amount of lemon juice.

3. Serve in bowls garnished with the tomato and parsley in the center. Refrigerate in airtight containers for up to 5 days or freeze without the parsley and tomato for up to 3 months.

TIP: If you find fava beans in tomato sauce, those are delicious in this recipe, too. Always rinse canned beans until there's no foam left to reduce the sodium and saponin content. The foam is created by saponins, which are antinutrients.

Per serving: Calories: 229; Total fat: 7.5g; Total carbs: 30g; Cholesterol: 0mg; Fiber: 8.5g; Sugar: 1.5g; Protein: 10g; Sodium: 806mg

LENTIL AND CARROT SALAD

Prep time: 10 minutes | **Cook time:** 20 minutes | **Makes** 4 servings

This is an ideal salad for meal prepping or potlucks. Inexpensive to make but very flavorful and healthy, it is also a perfect side dish for any meat entrée.

1 cup dried lentils, rinsed

2 medium carrots, diced into ¼- to ⅜-inch pieces

2 medium garlic cloves, minced

⅓ cup, plus 1 teaspoon olive oil, divided

2 tablespoons freshly squeezed lemon juice

½ teaspoon sea salt

⅛ teaspoon ground black pepper

3 large scallions, green parts only, diced

¼ cup chopped fresh flat-leaf parsley

2 ounces crumbled goat cheese (optional)

1. In a medium saucepan, combine the lentils, carrots, garlic, and 1 teaspoon of oil and cover with an inch of water. Cook over medium heat for 20 minutes, or until the lentils are tender but not mushy. Drain and set aside to cool.

2. In a small bowl, whisk together the remaining ⅓ cup of olive oil, lemon juice, salt, and pepper.

3. In a large bowl, combine the lentils, scallions, and parsley. Pour in the dressing and toss to coat the salad ingredients.

4. Serve at room temperature or chilled. Garnish with goat cheese (if using). Store in the refrigerator in an airtight container for up to 5 days or in the freezer for up to 3 months.

TIP: If you tolerate red onion and celery, consider adding ½ to 1 cup of each of those for variety. You can also serve this on a bed of greens.

Per serving: Calories: 338; Total fat: 20g; Total carbs: 31g; Cholesterol: 0mg; Fiber: 8.5g; Sugar: 2.5g; Protein: 11g; Sodium: 321mg

ORANGE, AVOCADO, AND JICAMA SALAD

Prep time: 10 minutes | **Makes** 3 servings

This is fast and easy to make anytime of the year. The orange segments, avocado, and jicama contribute to the variety of textures and depth of flavors in this year-round salad. If you're not familiar with jicama (pronounced HEE-kah-mah or HICK-ah-mah), you're in for a treat. It's crisp and crunchy like a radish and rich in prebiotic fiber, but ½ cup is considered low-FODMAP.

3 tablespoons avocado oil or olive oil

1 tablespoon champagne vinegar

¼ teaspoon sea salt

⅛ teaspoon ground black pepper

1 large orange, peeled and segmented

½ medium jicama, peeled and cut into matchsticks

1 small avocado, pitted, peeled, and cubed

¼ bunch fresh cilantro, chopped

1. In a small bowl or cup, whisk together the oil and vinegar. Season with the salt and pepper.

2. In a large bowl, combine the orange segments, jicama, avocado, and cilantro. Gently toss with the oil and vinegar mixture to combine and coat well.

3. This is best eaten right away, but it can be refrigerated in an airtight container and eaten within 1 day.

TIP: For a sweeter dressing, substitute freshly squeezed orange juice for the vinegar.

Per serving: Calories: 247; Total fat: 20g; Total carbs: 18g; Cholesterol: 0mg; Fiber: 9g; Sugar: 6g; Protein: 2g; Sodium: 202mg

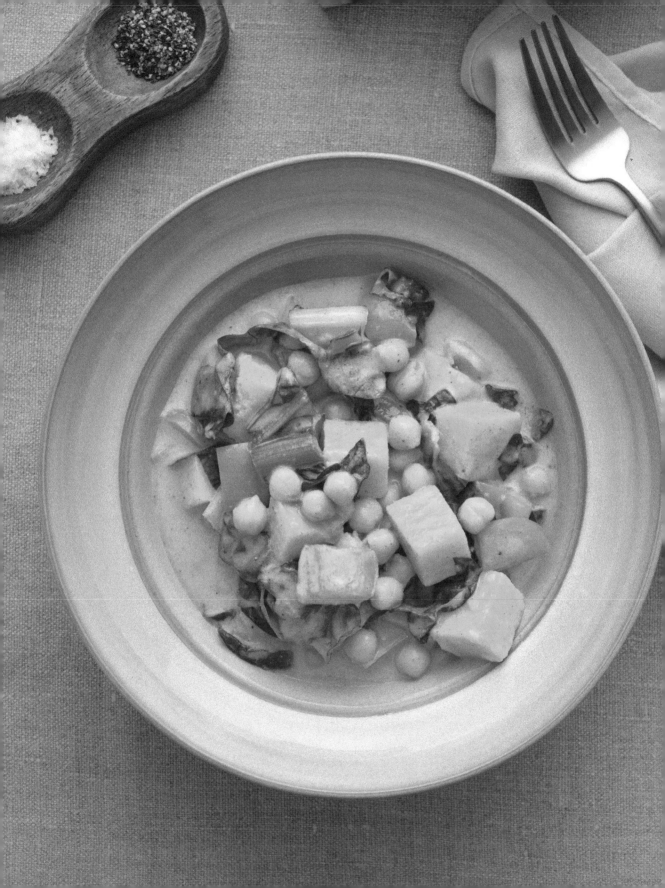

Chapter 4

MAINS

SCALLOPED ZUCCHINI WITH SHRIMP

Prep time: 15 minutes | **Cook time:** 30 minutes | **Makes** 4 servings

Shrimp turns an easy side dish into a delicious entrée. It's lighter and healthier than most scalloped dishes. This will be your go-to recipe when gardens are bursting with zucchini.

2 tablespoons Garlic Oil (page 115) or olive oil, plus more for greasing

4 medium zucchini, cut into ⅜-inch-thick slices

1 teaspoon sea salt, divided

2 tablespoons arrowroot starch/flour

¾ cup plain unsweetened almond milk

1 pound wild-caught medium/large shrimp, peeled and deveined

2 tablespoons chopped fresh chives

2 tablespoons chopped fresh flat-leaf parsley

¾ cup crushed Rice Flour Crackers (page 89) or gluten-free panko breadcrumbs

3 tablespoons ghee, butter, or substitute, melted

1. Preheat the oven to 350°F. Oil a 2-quart casserole dish and set aside.

2. Put the zucchini in a strainer. Sprinkle with ½ teaspoon of salt, tossing to combine. Set the strainer over a bowl to drain.

3. In a small saucepan, heat the garlic oil over medium-low heat. Mix in the arrowroot and the remaining ½ teaspoon of salt. Add the milk. Cook, stirring constantly, for about 3 minutes, until the sauce thickens and bubbles. Add the shrimp, chives, and parsley. Keep warm over low heat.

4. Layer the zucchini in the casserole dish. Spread the shrimp sauce over the zucchini.

5. In a small bowl, mix the crackers and ghee and sprinkle over the zucchini. Cover and bake for 25 minutes, or until the shrimp are firm and the zucchini is soft.

6. Serve hot. Refrigerate leftovers for up to 4 days or freeze for up to 3 months.

> **TIP:** After recovery, swap the zucchini for a higher-fiber vegetable like butternut squash or yams and cook for about 10 minutes longer.

Per serving: Calories: 415; Total fat: 26g; Total carbs: 24g; Cholesterol: 203mg; Fiber: 2g; Sugar: 5g; Protein: 23g; Sodium: 866mg

EASY PUMPKIN RISOTTO

Prep time: 10 minutes | **Cook time:** 25 minutes | **Makes** 6 servings

This dish comes together quickly using frozen vegetables, while the rice cooks in gut-healing bone broth. The Dijon adds a bit of tang without masking the natural flavors of the turkey, pumpkin, and spinach.

2 tablespoons Garlic Oil (page 115) or olive oil, divided

½ cup Arborio rice

¾ cup Chicken Bone Broth (page 114)

½ cup pumpkin puree

8 ounces frozen spinach, thawed

8 ounces ground turkey

2 teaspoons Dijon mustard

½ teaspoon sea salt

1. In a small saucepan, heat 1 tablespoon of the oil over medium-high heat. Add the rice and cook for 2 minutes, or until the rice starts to become translucent. Add the broth and pumpkin. Bring to a boil and cover; reduce the heat to medium-low. Simmer for about 20 minutes, until the liquid is fully absorbed and the rice is soft. Add more broth if needed. Add the spinach in the last 5 minutes.

2. Meanwhile, in a medium skillet, heat the remaining 1 tablespoon of oil over medium-high heat. Add the turkey, breaking it up, and cook for about 15 minutes, until it's light brown.

3. Add the turkey and Dijon to the saucepan. Stir to combine and season with the salt.

4. Serve immediately or store in an airtight container in the refrigerator for up to 4 days or in the freezer for up to 3 months.

> **TIP:** For variety, use butternut squash puree rather than pumpkin. Swap the turkey and spinach for chicken and other frozen greens such as collard greens, or add your favorite herbs and spices.

Per serving: Calories: 178; Total fat: 7.5g; Total carbs: 16g; Cholesterol: 27mg; Fiber: 2g; Sugar: 1g; Protein: 11g; Sodium: 324mg

MASHED POTATOES WITH CHICKEN GRAVY

Prep time: 15 minutes | **Cook time:** 20 minutes | **Makes** 3 servings

Mashed potatoes and gravy are good comfort food for recovery. This chicken gravy provides some protein and is also great over Herbed Rice Flour Biscuits (page 120). You'll have this on the table in just over 30 minutes, giving you time to steam some spinach to serve with it, if desired.

1 pound Yukon Gold potatoes, peeled and cut into 1-inch cubes

1 teaspoon sea salt, divided

2 tablespoons olive oil, divided

8 ounces ground chicken

2 teaspoons coconut aminos

2½ tablespoons arrowroot starch/flour

½ cup, plus 2 tablespoons Chicken Bone Broth (page 114), divided

½ cup plain unsweetened almond milk

1 teaspoon poultry seasoning

1. Place the potatoes in a large saucepan and cover them with cold water. Add ½ teaspoon of salt and bring to a boil over high heat. Lower the heat to medium and gently simmer for 18 to 20 minutes, or until the potatoes are completely tender when pierced with a fork.

2. Meanwhile, in a small skillet over medium heat, heat 1 tablespoon of olive oil. Add the ground chicken and cook for about 5 minutes, stirring frequently. Add the coconut aminos and cook for about 2 more minutes, until the chicken is crumbly and cooked through.

3. In a small bowl or glass measuring cup, whisk the arrowroot with ½ cup of the broth and the milk. Pour the mixture over the chicken and stir to combine. Cook over medium heat, stirring constantly, for about 3 minutes, until the gravy thickens. Do not boil the arrowroot, or it will be gummy. Season with the poultry seasoning and the remaining ½ teaspoon of salt. Reduce the heat to low to keep the dish warm.

4. When the potatoes are done cooking, drain them, leaving a little of the starchy liquid in the pan. Add the remaining 1 tablespoon of olive oil and mash the potatoes well with a potato masher or electric mixer. Add the remaining 2 tablespoons of broth, if needed, to reach your desired consistency.

5. Serve the gravy over the mashed potatoes. Store any leftovers in airtight containers in the refrigerator for up to 4 days or in the freezer for up to 3 months.

TIP: For creamier gravy, use 1 cup of almond milk and no broth. If you have leftover ground chicken, add some Breakfast Sausage Seasoning (page 116) and cook or freeze it.

Per serving: Calories: 312; Total fat: 10g; Total carbs: 34g; Cholesterol: 44mg; Fiber: 3g; Sugar: 2g; Protein: 22g; Sodium: 679mg

RICE-CRUSTED SPINACH QUICHE

Prep time: 15 minutes | **Cook time:** 30 minutes | **Makes** 4 servings

This gluten-free, dairy-free quiche is super easy to make compliant with the Low-Fiber Phase. Enjoy it for breakfast, lunch, or dinner.

1⅓ cups cooked Arborio rice

1 tablespoon coconut oil

5 large eggs, divided

2 tablespoons arrowroot starch/flour

1½ tablespoons nutritional yeast

1 tablespoon Dijon mustard

1 tablespoon freshly squeezed lemon juice

1 teaspoon sea salt

2¼ cups plain unsweetened almond milk

8 ounces frozen spinach, thawed

1. Preheat the oven to 400°F. Oil a 9-inch pie plate with the coconut oil and set aside.

2. In a large mixing bowl, beat 1 egg. Mix in the rice. Transfer the mixture to the pie plate. With the back of a spoon, press the rice into the bottom and sides of the plate to form a crust.

3. In the same mixing bowl, beat 1 egg with an electric hand mixer until frothy. Add the arrowroot and beat well. Add the remaining 3 eggs. Beat for about 3 minutes, or until the mixture is light and frothy. Add the nutritional yeast, Dijon, lemon juice, and salt. Beat for 2 minutes while gradually adding the milk.

4. Squeeze the spinach to drain it, then add it to the mixing bowl and stir to combine.

5. Gently pour the egg mixture on top of the rice crust. Bake for 30 minutes, or until the top is golden and a knife inserted in the center comes out clean. Cool for 10 minutes before cutting.

6. Serve, or refrigerate in an airtight container for up to 4 days or freeze for up to 3 months.

TIP: Add your favorite ingredients, like sautéed onions, bell pepper, mushrooms, olives, and/or shredded dairy-free cheese.

Per serving: Calories: 267; Total fat: 11g; Total carbs: 26g; Cholesterol: 232mg; Fiber: 2.5g; Sugar: 0.5g; Protein: 13g; Sodium: 910mg

SALMON AND GREEN PEAS WITH GARLIC-GINGER SAUCE

Prep time: 10 minutes | **Cook time:** 20 minutes | **Makes** 4 servings

This recipe isn't just fast and easy but also healthy and high-fiber. The ginger, garlic, orange, and sesame sauce flavors top it all off with rich, savory deliciousness.

1 tablespoon olive oil

4 (6-ounce) salmon fillets

¼ teaspoon sea salt

12 ounces frozen green peas

2 cups cooked brown rice

½ cup Garlic-Ginger Sauce (page 118)

1. Preheat the oven to 400°F. Line a baking sheet with parchment paper.

2. Drizzle the oil over the salmon fillets and season them with the salt. Add the salmon to the baking sheet and bake for 17 minutes, or until the salmon reaches 145°F and flakes easily with a fork.

3. Cook the peas in the microwave or in a steamer over boiling water for about 5 minutes. Add the rice to the steamer with the peas.

4. Serve the rice and peas topped with a salmon fillet and drizzled with the garlic-ginger sauce. Store leftovers in an airtight container in the refrigerator for up to 3 days or in the freezer up to 3 months.

TIP: If you don't have the garlic-ginger sauce, you can use a gluten-free teriyaki or other sauce.

Per serving: Calories: 560; Total fat: 21g; Total carbs: 44g; Cholesterol: 107mg; Fiber: 5.5g; Sugar: 7.5g; Protein: 47g; Sodium: 845mg

ARTICHOKE AND SHRIMP PASTA

Prep time: 15 minutes | **Cook time:** 15 minutes | **Makes** 5 servings

Artichokes and shrimp are the perfect combo in this fast, easy dish. The parsley and wine add to the richness, while the lentil pasta and artichokes boost the fiber content and the bone broth provides gut-healing amino acids.

12 ounces lentil pasta

3 tablespoons arrowroot starch/ flour

1 cup Chicken Bone Broth (page 114)

2 tablespoons Garlic Oil (page 115) or olive oil

1 pound wild-caught jumbo shrimp, peeled and deveined

1 teaspoon sea salt, divided

16 ounces artichoke hearts, quartered (water-packed or frozen and thawed)

½ cup dry white wine (optional)

2 tablespoons chopped fresh flat-leaf parsley

⅛ teaspoon ground black pepper

1. Bring a large pot of water to a boil over high heat. Cook the pasta according to the package directions (usually 10 to 15 minutes).

2. Meanwhile, in a small bowl, whisk the arrowroot into the broth. Set aside.

3. In a large skillet, heat the oil over medium-high heat. Put the shrimp in the skillet. Season with ½ teaspoon of salt and cook for 2 minutes; flip and cook for 1 minute, until the shrimp starts to firm up.

4. Add the arrowroot mixture and artichoke hearts. Cook for 5 to 7 minutes, stirring frequently, until the mixture thickens. Stir in the wine (if using) and parsley. Cook for 5 minutes over medium heat until the wine is reduced. Season with the remaining ½ teaspoon of salt and the pepper.

5. Drain the pasta and toss it with the sauce. Serve promptly or cool and refrigerate in an airtight container for up to 4 days.

TIP: Most stores carry lentil pasta. Use chickpea if you can't find lentil, or check the Resources (see page 130) for where to buy the pasta.

Per serving: Calories: 420; Total fat: 7g; Total carbs: 52g; Cholesterol: 109mg; Fiber: 6.5g; Sugar: 0g; Protein: 33g; Sodium: 1,108mg

ASIAN-INSPIRED TURKEY LOAF

Prep time: 10 minutes | **Cook time:** 35 minutes | **Makes** 4 servings

This isn't your typical meat loaf. The sesame, ginger, and five-spice powder add a delicious Asian flair, while the navy beans contribute fiber. To complete the menu, this meat loaf would be great with a baked sweet potato and/or Green Beans with Garlic-Ginger Sauce (page 91).

3 tablespoons coconut aminos

1 tablespoon olive oil

1 teaspoon sesame oil

5 large scallions, green parts only, thinly sliced

2 tablespoons ground flaxseed

1 (1-inch) piece fresh ginger, peeled and finely grated

¾ teaspoon five-spice powder

1 (15-ounce) can navy beans, rinsed and drained

1 pound ground turkey

1. Preheat the oven to 375°F. Line a baking sheet with parchment paper and set aside.

2. In a large bowl, whisk together the coconut aminos, olive oil, and sesame oil. Add the scallions, flaxseed, ginger, and five-spice powder.

3. Put the beans on a cutting board or other flat surface and mash them with a potato masher until no whole beans remain. Add the beans and turkey to the bowl and stir to mix.

4. Shape the mixture into a loaf and place it on the prepared baking sheet. Bake for about 35 minutes, or until the turkey loaf has reached an internal temperature of 165°F.

5. Serve hot or store in an airtight container in the refrigerator for up to 5 days or in the freezer for up to 3 months.

> **TIP:** To bake sweet potatoes for serving with the meat loaf, slice them in half vertically, spray them with olive oil, and put them cut-side down on the baking sheet. They will be fork-tender in 30 to 35 minutes.

Per serving: Calories: 372; Total fat: 15g; Total carbs: 28g; Cholesterol: 78mg; Fiber: 7g; Sugar: 3g; Protein: 32g; Sodium: 656mg

SALMON AND BEAN LOAF

Prep time: 15 minutes | **Cook time:** 40 minutes | **Makes** 4 servings

In this salmon loaf, canned salmon provides flavor while oats and navy beans provide fiber at a budget-friendly price. I snuck in a carrot and some scallions for a little extra fiber and flavor to complement the lemon and Dijon.

1 tablespoon coconut oil

¾ cup gluten-free rolled oats

3 large eggs, beaten

¼ cup mayonnaise

Juice of 1 small lemon

1 teaspoon Dijon mustard

½ teaspoon sea salt

1 (15-ounce) can low-sodium small white beans, rinsed, drained, and mashed

1 (5-ounce) can water-packed wild-caught salmon, drained

1 large carrot, shredded

2 large scallions, green parts only, chopped

1. Preheat the oven to 375°F. Grease a 9 x 5 x 3-inch loaf pan with the coconut oil and set aside.

2. In a blender, process the oats on medium speed just until they are powdery.

3. In a large bowl, whisk together the eggs, mayonnaise, lemon juice, Dijon, and salt.

4. Add the mashed beans, salmon, carrot, and scallions to the large bowl and mix with your hands, flaking the salmon and disbursing the ingredients evenly throughout. Spread the mixture out evenly in the prepared loaf pan. Bake for 40 minutes, until the center is set.

5. Serve hot or cold and store in an airtight container in the refrigerator for up to 4 days or in the freezer for up to 3 months.

TIP: If desired, serve with your favorite tartar sauce, cocktail sauce, or hot white cream sauce. Consider serving with steamed snow peas or roasted asparagus.

Per serving: Calories: 373; Total fat: 20g; Total carbs: 31g; Cholesterol: 158mg; Fiber: 7.5g; Sugar: 2.5g; Protein: 19g; Sodium: 1,085mg

CHICKEN ENCHILADAS

Prep time: 15 minutes | **Cook time:** 30 minutes | **Makes** 6 servings

This yummy sauce takes enchiladas to a new level. Flavorful tomatillo Salsa Verde is blended with cashew sour cream to create a creamy, rich fiesta in your mouth. The avocados add more creamy richness and fiber.

1 tablespoon coconut oil

1 cup cashews, soaked overnight and drained

½ cup filtered water

2 tablespoons freshly squeezed lime juice

2½ cups Salsa Verde (page 123), divided

3 cups Tender Stewed Chicken, shredded (page 117)

12 medium corn tortillas

1 large ripe avocado, pitted, peeled, and sliced

4 medium scallions, green parts only, thinly sliced

1. Preheat the oven to 375°F. Grease a 13 x 9-inch casserole dish with the oil and set aside.

2. In a food processor or blender, blend the cashews, water, and lime juice until smooth. Add 1½ cups of the salsa verde and blend well. Coat the bottom of the casserole dish with a ladle of the sauce. Transfer the remaining mixture to a large shallow bowl and set aside.

3. In a medium bowl, mix the remaining 1 cup of salsa verde with the chicken.

4. Dip each tortilla into the bowl with the sauce to lightly coat. Spoon ¼ cup of the chicken mixture into each tortilla. Roll and place each one seam-side down in the casserole dish. Top with the remaining sauce. Bake for 25 to 30 minutes, until bubbly.

5. Serve garnished with the avocado and scallions, or store ungarnished in an airtight container in the refrigerator for up to 5 days or in the freezer for up to 3 months.

TIP: You can use your favorite enchilada sauce for these, but be sure to read the ingredients.

Per serving (2 enchiladas): Calories: 639; Total fat: 28g; Total carbs: 44g; Cholesterol: 134mg; Fiber: 8g; Sugar: 9.5g; Protein: 52g; Sodium: 1,151mg

SPAGHETTI SQUASH WITH CLAM SAUCE

Prep time: 15 minutes | **Cook time:** 45 minutes | **Makes** 3 servings

This dish deliciously blends the mild taste of spaghetti squash with the salty sweetness of clams. Spaghetti squash is a great alternative to grain pasta for your favorite sauces. It is high in fiber and essential vitamins, and low in calories and carbs. The clams contribute protein and vitamins C, B_2, and B_{12}, along with iron, potassium, iodine, selenium, and anti-inflammatory omega-3 fatty acids.

1 medium spaghetti squash

3 tablespoons Garlic Oil (page 115) or olive oil, divided

½ teaspoon sea salt, divided

1 tablespoon arrowroot starch/flour

1 teaspoon lemon zest

Pinch ground white pepper

1 (6½-ounce) can chopped clams

½ cup dry white wine (optional)

½ cup vegetable broth or Chicken Bone Broth (page 114)

3 tablespoons chopped fresh flat-leaf parsley leaves

1. Preheat the oven to 400°F. Line a baking sheet with parchment paper and set aside.

2. Halve the squash lengthwise and scrape the seeds out. Brush or spray the cut sides with 1 tablespoon of oil and sprinkle with ¼ teaspoon of the salt.

3. Bake in the oven, cut-side down, for 35 to 45 minutes, until the squash is soft when poked with a fork.

4. Meanwhile, in a medium saucepan, heat the remaining 2 tablespoons of oil over medium heat. Quickly stir in the arrowroot, lemon zest, the remaining ¼ teaspoon of salt, and the white pepper, stirring constantly. Drain the juice from the clams into the pan, setting the clams aside. Reduce the heat to low. Stir the wine (if using) and broth into the pan and continue stirring for about 5 minutes, until the mixture thickens and bubbles or until the wine is reduced. Stir in the clams and let them heat through for 1 to 2 minutes.

5. Remove the squash from the oven. Carefully scoop out the "spaghetti" and portion it onto serving plates or cool and put in storage containers. Top with the sauce and sprinkle with parsley. Serve immediately, or store leftovers in an airtight container in the refrigerator for up to 3 days or in the freezer up to 2 months.

> **TIP:** If desired, use 1 pound of fresh, scrubbed clams instead of canned. Discard any with broken shells. Soak the clams in 2 quarts of water and 3 tablespoons of sea salt for 20 minutes. Discard any floaters. Scrub the clams again. Steam for 5 to 7 minutes in 1 inch of water until they open. Discard any that don't open. Use ½ cup of the steaming water in the sauce. Leave the clams in their shells for serving.

Per serving: Calories: 324; Total fat: 16g; Total carbs: 43g; Cholesterol: 5mg; Fiber: 8g; Sugar: 15g; Protein: 6g; Sodium: 928mg

DILL AND LIMA BEAN RICE WITH CHICKEN

Prep time: 10 minutes | **Cook time:** 55 minutes | **Makes** 4 servings

This dish was inspired by another of my favorite Persian dishes that takes hours to make. I drastically reduced the time, changed the rice to brown rice, and used chicken thighs instead of lamb shanks. It's great for meal prepping and can be eaten hot or cold. The dill makes this dish scrumptious.

2 tablespoons olive oil

1 large onion, cut vertically into slivers

2 cups Chicken Bone Broth (page 114)

16 ounces frozen lima beans

⅔ cup brown rice

3 tablespoons dried dill weed

½ teaspoon sea salt

⅛ teaspoon ground black pepper

4 large bone-in chicken thighs

1. Preheat the oven to 375°F.

2. In a large oven-proof Dutch oven, heat the oil over medium heat. Sauté the onion for 5 minutes, or until it is soft and translucent.

3. Add the broth and bring to a boil. Add the lima beans and rice and bring to a boil again. Stir in the dill weed, salt, and pepper. Arrange the chicken on top.

4. Bake for 45 minutes, until the chicken reaches 165°F and the rice is done.

5. Enjoy right away or store in airtight containers in the refrigerator for up to 4 days or in the freezer for up to 3 months.

TIP: To kick it up a notch, add red pepper flakes to taste.

Per serving: Calories: 619; Total fat: 27g; Total carbs: 57g; Cholesterol: 116mg; Fiber: 9g; Sugar: 2g; Protein: 35g; Sodium: 603mg

CURRIED CHICKPEA STEW

Prep time: 15 minutes | **Cook time:** 25 minutes | **Makes** 4 servings

Your house will smell heavenly when you cook this aromatic stew. Packed with fiber-rich chickpeas and vegetables, this stew satisfies so much that you won't miss the meat. It's great for meal prepping and freezing.

3 tablespoons arrowroot starch/flour

2 cups full-fat coconut milk

1 tablespoon curry powder

2 tablespoons olive oil

1 (2-inch) piece fresh ginger, peeled and grated or minced

1 pound Swiss chard (leaves and stems), chopped

1 medium sweet potato, peeled and cut into 1-inch cubes

1 large red bell pepper, roughly chopped

¾ teaspoon sea salt

½ teaspoon ground black pepper

1 (15-ounce) can chickpeas, drained and rinsed

1. In a small bowl, whisk the arrowroot into the coconut milk until there are no clumps remaining. Whisk in the curry powder until it is thoroughly blended. Set aside.

2. In a large Dutch oven, heat the oil over medium-high heat until hot but not smoking. Sauté the ginger for about 2 minutes. Add the coconut milk mixture, chard stems, sweet potato, and bell pepper. Season with the salt and pepper. Bring to a boil, then reduce the heat to medium and simmer for 10 minutes. Add the chard leaves and simmer 2 to 5 minutes longer, until the sweet potato is softened.

3. Stir in the chickpeas and let them heat up for a few minutes in the stew before serving.

4. Serve in bowls, or cool and refrigerate for up to 4 days or freeze for up to 3 months in an airtight container.

TIP: For variety, add parsley at the end, and instead of curry powder (I prefer Madras curry powder), use Moroccan rub, garam masala, or berbere. Red pepper flakes add a nice zing.

Per serving: Calories: 455; Total fat: 33g; Total carbs: 36g; Cholesterol: 0mg; Fiber: 9g; Sugar: 6.5g; Protein: 9g; Sodium: 834mg

PERSIAN-INSPIRED RICE AND BEANS

Prep time: 15 minutes | **Cook time:** 30 minutes | **Makes** 3 servings

The flavors and plentiful, vibrant herbs and greens in my favorite Persian stew, *gormeh sabzi*, were the inspiration for this dish. There's no fenugreek, so add 1 to 2 teaspoons, if desired. Authentic Persian dishes can take hours to prepare, but this one is done in under an hour.

2 tablespoons olive oil

5 ounces baby spinach

1 bunch fresh flat-leaf parsley, large stems removed, chopped

4 large scallions, green parts only, chopped

¾ cup Chicken Bone Broth (page 114)

1 medium lime, zested and juiced

1 tablespoon pure maple syrup

½ teaspoon ground mustard

½ teaspoon curry powder

¼ teaspoon sea salt

1 (15-ounce) can kidney beans, drained and rinsed

1½ cups cooked brown rice

1. In a medium Dutch oven, heat the olive oil over medium-high heat. Add the spinach, parsley, and scallions. Cook, stirring frequently for 10 minutes.

2. Add the broth, lime juice and zest, maple syrup, mustard, curry powder, and salt. Bring to a rolling boil. Reduce the heat to low. Cover and cook for 15 minutes. Stir in the beans and rice; let them heat through for about 2 minutes.

3. Serve while hot or cool and refrigerate for up to 5 days or freeze for up to 3 months in an airtight container.

TIP: For lamb stew, add 12 ounces of lamb stew meat and 1 bay leaf with the broth. Simmer for at least 1 hour. Serve over the rice rather than mixing in the rice.

Per serving: Calories: 377; Total fat: 10g; Total carbs: 55g; Cholesterol: 1mg; Fiber: 9g; Sugar: 4.5g; Protein: 15g; Sodium: 593mg

ROASTED CHICKEN STRIPS AND ROOT VEGETABLES

Prep time: 15 minutes | **Cook time:** 35 minutes | **Makes** 3 servings

This sheet pan meal is a feast for the mouth and eyes. The colorful vegetables pack a load of fiber, as does the chicken's cracker-and-flaxseed coating.

½ cup plain unsweetened almond milk

½ teaspoon vinegar

13 ounces chicken thighs, cut into 1½-inch-wide strips

12 ounces parsnips, cut diagonally (¼ inch thick)

12 ounces rainbow carrots, cut diagonally (¼ inch thick)

2 tablespoons olive oil

1 teaspoon sea salt, divided

¾ cup finely crushed Rice Flour Crackers (page 89) or almond flour

2 tablespoons ground flaxseed

1 teaspoon Italian seasoning

100 percent olive oil cooking spray

1. Preheat the oven to 400°F. Line 1 large and 1 small baking sheet with parchment paper.

2. In a large shallow bowl, combine the milk and vinegar. Add the chicken strips to soak.

3. Arrange the parsnips and carrots on the large baking sheet. Drizzle with the olive oil and sprinkle with ½ teaspoon of salt. Toss to coat, then spread the vegetables out.

4. In another shallow bowl, mix the cracker crumbs, flaxseed, Italian seasoning, and the remaining ½ teaspoon of salt.

5. Dip each chicken strip in the cracker mixture, then arrange them on the small baking sheet. Spray the chicken lightly with cooking spray. Bake for 35 minutes, or until the chicken is cooked through to 165°F and the vegetables are fork-tender. After 20 minutes, flip the chicken and stir the vegetables.

6. Serve, or refrigerate for up to 4 days or freeze for up to 3 months in an airtight container.

TIP: Chicken thighs tend to be less dry than breasts.

Per serving: Calories: 612; Total fat: 37g; Total carbs: 51g; Cholesterol: 139mg; Fiber: 9.5g; Sugar: 11g; Protein: 25g; Sodium: 822mg

BEET AND LENTIL BOWL

Prep time: 15 minutes | **Cook time:** 10 minutes | **Makes** 2 servings

This is a dish that's both pretty and delicious. If you can tolerate it, a bed of baby kale and a sprinkle of red pepper flakes would also be superb. If you can't find red lentils, use another color or drained and rinsed canned lentils.

½ cup red lentils, rinsed and drained

1¼ cups Chicken Bone Broth (page 114)

½ teaspoon sea salt (optional)

2 large eggs

¼ cup Savory Sauce and Dip (page 122)

1 cup canned beets (not pickled), cut in cubes

1 small avocado, pitted, peeled, and diced

¼ cup roasted sunflower seeds

1. In a small saucepan, bring the lentils and broth to a boil. Cover and reduce the heat to a simmer for about 8 minutes, or until the lentils are tender. Drain any excess liquid and add the salt (if using).

2. In another small saucepan, cover the eggs with cold water. Bring to a boil over medium-high heat. Lower the heat to a simmer and cook for 7 minutes. Rinse the eggs under cold running water, then peel and halve them lengthwise.

3. If the sauce has been refrigerated and has thickened, warm it slightly for a few seconds in the microwave or in a saucepan over low heat for 1 to 2 minutes.

4. To assemble, spread the lentils over the bottom of a bowl. Top each bowl with the beets, avocado, 2 tablespoons of sauce, 2 egg halves, and garnish with sunflower seeds.

5. Serve, or store leftovers in an airtight container in the refrigerator and enjoy cold the next day.

TIP: To toast raw sunflower seeds, spray or drizzle them with olive oil, sprinkle with salt, and toast them in a toaster oven or in the oven on broil for about 3 minutes until lightly toasted.

Per serving: Calories: 548; Total fat: 29g; Total carbs: 47g; Cholesterol: 189mg; Fiber: 12g; Sugar: 5.5g; Protein: 30g; Sodium: 620mg

CHICKPEA PASTA WITH PUMPKIN SEED PESTO

Prep time: 10 minutes | **Cook time:** 15 minutes | **Makes** 4 servings

This fast, easy dish is so delicious, it might become one of your go-to meals. Chickpeas are powerhouses for plant-based protein and fiber, so chickpea pasta is a great alternative to grain-based pasta.

1⅓ cups sliced carrots (⅛ inch thick)

1½ cups chopped broccoli

8 ounces chickpea pasta

½ cup pumpkin seeds

2 garlic cloves, peeled

¾ cup fresh basil

¾ cup fresh flat-leaf parsley

2 tablespoons freshly squeezed lemon juice

1 teaspoon sea salt

½ cup olive oil

1. In a large pot that fits a steamer basket or insert, bring 1 inch of water to a boil. Put the carrots into the steamer basket in the pot. Cover the pot and cook for 5 minutes. Add the broccoli and cook for 5 to 8 minutes, until the vegetables are as tender as you prefer.

2. Cook the pasta according to the package instructions until soft.

3. Meanwhile, in a food processor or blender, pulse the pumpkin seeds and garlic for about 20 seconds, until the seeds are almost ground. Add the basil, parsley, lemon juice, and salt. While processing, slowly stream in the oil until the mixture resembles a coarse paste.

4. When the pasta is done, drain it and toss it with the vegetables and pesto. Serve or cool and refrigerate in an airtight container for up to 4 days, including the time since the pesto was made. I don't recommend freezing it.

TIP: To save time when prepping dinner, make and refrigerate the pesto up to 4 days in advance.

Per serving: Calories: 598; Total fat: 39g; Total carbs: 46g; Cholesterol: 0mg; Fiber: 12g; Sugar: 5g; Protein: 19g; Sodium: 634mg

SOUTHWESTERN GRITS BOWL

Prep time: 15 minutes | **Cook time:** 10 minutes | **Makes** 3 servings

Who says grits are only for breakfast? Grits provide the base for this bowl, which makes a fast, easy breakfast, lunch, or dinner. The grits, beans, and avocado team up to provide a big boost of fiber while the green chiles and Tex-Mex Seasoning provide a big boost of flavor.

1 cup plain unsweetened almond milk

¾ cup filtered water, divided

½ cup regular grits (not instant)

1 (4-ounce) can diced green chiles

1 (15-ounce) can black beans, rinsed and drained

1½ teaspoons Tex-Mex Seasoning (page 121) or ground cumin

1 small avocado, pitted, peeled, and diced

1 small lime, cut into wedges

1. In a medium saucepan, bring the milk and ½ cup of water to a boil over medium-high heat. Whisk in the grits and green chiles and their juices. Cover and cook 5 to 7 minutes, or until all the liquid has been absorbed.

2. In a large skillet, combine the beans, Tex-Mex seasoning, and remaining ¼ cup of water over medium heat. Cook for 4 to 5 minutes, or until the liquid is nearly evaporated.

3. Serve the grits topped with the beans and avocado, and garnish with lime wedges for squeezing over the dish. Store any leftover beans and grits in airtight containers and refrigerate for up to 4 days. Add the avocado and lime wedges when serving.

TIP: See Resources (see page 130) for where to buy regular gluten-free grits.

Per serving: Calories: 331; Total fat: 8.5g; Total carbs: 52g; Cholesterol: 0mg; Fiber: 14g; Sugar: 2g; Protein: 13g; Sodium: 827mg

TEX-MEX FLATBREADS

Prep time: 10 minutes | **Cook time:** 15 minutes | **Makes** 4 servings

Having the flatbreads made in advance helps put this meal together quickly, so you might want to make and freeze some flatbreads to have on hand. In this dish, walnuts provide plant-based protein and a meaty texture to absorb the Tex-Mex Seasoning. These little flatbreads are very filling and satisfying.

4 flatbreads from Grain-Free Baguette, Rolls, or Flatbreads (page 124)

¾ cup walnut pieces, finely chopped

1½ tablespoons water

½ teaspoon Tex-Mex Seasoning (page 121)

½ cup Salsa Verde (page 123)

1 medium tomato, diced

2 small avocados, pitted, peeled, and diced

¼ cup chopped fresh cilantro

1. Preheat the oven to 400°F.

2. Put the flatbreads on a baking sheet or baking stone.

3. In a small bowl, mix the walnuts, water, and Tex-Mex seasoning.

4. Spread about 2 tablespoons of the salsa on each flatbread, then add 2 tablespoons of the walnuts, followed by 2 tablespoons of the diced tomato. Bake for 15 minutes.

5. Serve topped with avocado and cilantro. For meal prep storage, assemble the flatbreads up to the point of baking and refrigerate them in an airtight container for up to 4 days. I don't recommend refreezing the bread or freezing it with any toppings.

TIP: You can swap your favorite pizza crust for the flatbreads, packaged taco seasoning for the Tex-Mex Seasoning, and your favorite salsa for the Salsa Verde. Check the labels for ingredients and fiber.

Per serving: Calories: 563; Total fat: 38g; Total carbs: 45g; Cholesterol: 0mg; Fiber: 20g; Sugar: 6.5g; Protein: 17g; Sodium: 682mg

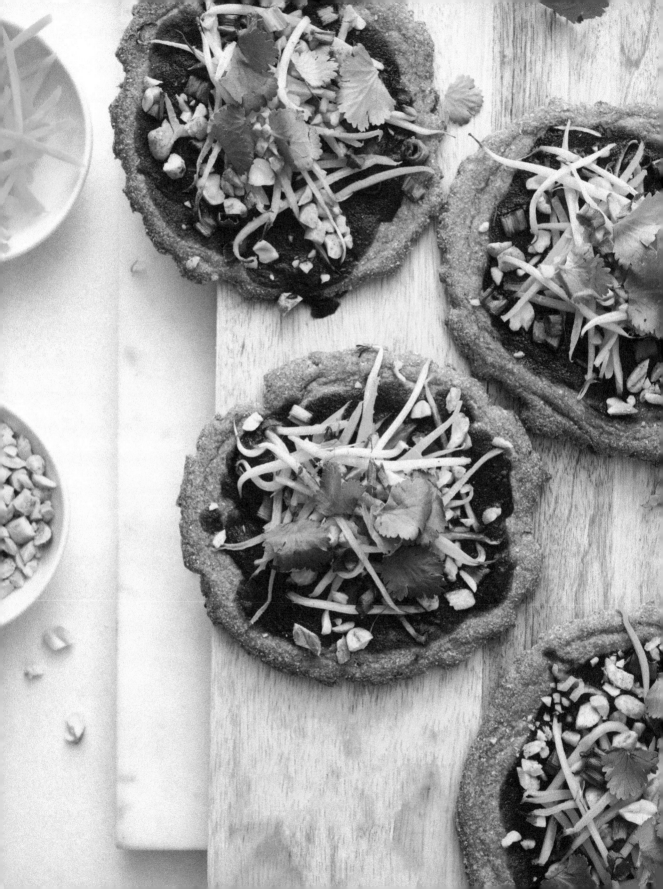

Chapter 5

SNACKS AND SIDES

LICORICE ICE POPS

Prep time: 10 minutes, plus 3 hours to freeze | **Cook time:** 5 minutes
Makes 3 servings

Ice pops make clear liquids more fun to consume. These ice pops are made with licorice root tea. Licorice root is 50 times sweeter than sugar and has numerous medicinal properties. It's often used to relieve an upset stomach or acid reflux and contains over 300 flavonoids with antiviral and antibacterial activity. Paired with coconut water for electrolytes, these ice pops will have you feeling better in no time.

½ cup filtered water
1½ teaspoons unflavored gelatin, preferably grass-fed
3 licorice root tea bags
1 cup coconut water

1. In a small saucepan, bring the water to a boil. Remove from the heat and add the gelatin, stirring until the gelatin is dissolved.

2. Add the tea bags and let the tea steep for 10 minutes.

3. Add the coconut water and stir to combine.

4. Pour the mixture into ice pop molds, leaving about ⅛ inch of headspace for expansion. Freeze the ice pops for at least 3 hours before eating. These will keep in the freezer for up to 3 months.

TIP: I recommend gelatin from grass-fed cows such as Great Lakes, if possible, but use what you can find. For popsicle molds, I use BPA-free ½-cup molds. If you don't have molds, you can use popsicle bags (see Resources, page 130) or paper cups with kraft sticks inserted halfway through freezing.

Per serving (1 ice pop): Calories: 16; Total fat: 0g; Total carbs: 4g; Cholesterol: 0mg; Fiber: 0g; Sugar: 3.5g; Protein: 0g; Sodium: 23mg

FRUIT PUNCH GELATIN JIGGLERS

Prep time: 10 minutes, plus 2 hours to chill | **Cook time:** 5 minutes
Makes 6 servings

Gelatin jigglers are delightful snacks. I threw tart cherry juice into the mix for its antioxidant and anti-inflammatory properties and because it is an excellent source of potassium and a rich source of vitamins and minerals. Its anthocyanins are what help reduce inflammation in arthritis and reduce uric acid in gout.

½ cup filtered water

2 tablespoons unflavored gelatin, preferably grass-fed

¾ cup unsweetened grape juice

¾ cup unsweetened filtered apple juice

½ cup 100 percent tart cherry juice

1. In a small saucepan, bring the water to a boil over high heat. Remove the pan from the heat and stir in the gelatin until the gelatin is completely dissolved. Set the mixture aside to cool.

2. In a medium bowl or dish, mix the grape, apple, and cherry juices together. Add the water and gelatin mixture. Stir well until the gelatin is fully incorporated.

3. Chill in the refrigerator for about 2 hours, or until set. Cut into squares or desired shapes, or just scoop into bowls.

4. Store in an airtight container in the refrigerator for 7 to 10 days. I don't recommend freezing unless you plan on eating these as a cold treat straight out of the freezer. The gelatin won't freeze solid, and they may turn slushy when thawed.

TIP: You can use a premixed fruit punch or any combination of allowable juices to make these.

Per serving: Calories: 44; Total fat: 0g; Total carbs: 11g; Cholesterol: 0mg; Fiber: 0g; Sugar: 10g; Protein: 0g; Sodium: 10mg

TURKEY-MAYO ROLL-UPS

Prep time: 5 minutes | **Makes** 3 servings

These are one of my favorite grab-and-go items for a quick, easy snack or lunch box element. Using 1½-ounce turkey slices, one serving is two roll-ups. Add your favorite herbs to the mayonnaise, if desired. For more fiber in the High-Fiber Phase, swap ready-made or Lima Bean Hummus with Pine Nuts (page 90) for the mayonnaise and consider adding roasted red pepper, slivered scallions, and/or fresh basil on top before rolling.

6 thin slices turkey breast (9 ounces total)

4½ tablespoons mayonnaise (see Tip)

1. On a clean work surface, lay out the turkey slices. Divide the mayonnaise between the slices and spread it around.

2. Starting at one end, roll each slice up tightly and secure with a toothpick.

TIP: To avoid unhealthy oils in commercial mayonnaise, whip up your own quickly by blending 1 large egg, 2 tablespoons of apple cider vinegar, and 1 teaspoon of sea salt in a blender or food processor on high. Very, very slowly stream in 1 cup of olive oil while continuing to blend. This makes about 1½ cups and can be stored in the refrigerator for up to 7 days. If you're concerned about raw egg and/or want the mayonnaise to keep for up to 1 month, use a pasteurized liquid egg product.

Per serving (2 roll-ups): Calories: 226; Total fat: 17g; Total carbs: 2g; Cholesterol: 51mg; Fiber: 0g; Sugar: 2g; Protein: 14g; Sodium: 915mg

RICE FLOUR CRACKERS

Prep time: 15 minutes | **Cook time:** 20 minutes | **Makes** 126 crackers

These crackers are great snacks in the Low-Fiber Phase and can be stored in an airtight container in a cool, dry place for up to 2 months. Feel free to add 1 or 2 teaspoons of your favorite seasoning, such as rosemary, Italian seasoning, or garlic powder, if tolerated.

2 cups Low-Fiber Flour Blend (page 119), plus more for dusting

1 teaspoon baking powder

½ teaspoon sea salt, plus more for sprinkling

½ cup cold ghee, plus 2 tablespoons melted ghee for brushing

⅔ cup plain unsweetened almond milk

1. Preheat the oven to 400°F. Cut 2 pieces of parchment paper to fit baking sheets and set aside.

2. In a large mixing bowl, mix the flour, baking powder, and salt. Cut the ½ cup of cold ghee into the flour until only small particles remain. Add the milk and mix until smooth. Form into 2 equal balls.

3. Lightly flour the prepared parchment pieces and roll a ball out on each to a $^1/_{16}$-inch-thick rectangle, about 11 × 14 inches. Dust the rolling pin and your hands with flour as needed to handle the dough. Using a table knife or pizza cutter, cut the rolled dough balls into a grid of 9 rows by 7 columns for crackers about 1½ inches square. Gently poke each cracker a couple times with a fork.

4. Transfer the dough on the parchment paper to baking sheets and bake for 20 minutes, or until golden and starting to crisp. Transfer the crackers on the parchment paper to a cooling rack. Brush with the melted ghee and sprinkle with salt.

TIP: You can mix the dough in a food processor.

Per serving (14 crackers): Calories: 245; Total fat: 15g; Total carbs: 27g; Cholesterol: 36mg; Fiber: 0.5g; Sugar: 0g; Protein: 1g; Sodium: 211mg

LIMA BEAN HUMMUS WITH PINE NUTS

Prep time: 10 minutes | **Cook time:** 20 minutes | **Makes** 1½ cups

This hummus is great served with raw vegetables or crackers like Rice Flour Crackers (page 89). Using pine nuts instead of tahini gives this dish a Mediterranean vibe. Pistachios would also be a delicious variation.

8 ounces frozen baby lima beans

2 tablespoons raw pine nuts

2 tablespoons freshly squeezed lemon juice

2 tablespoons dried dill weed

1 garlic clove, peeled

½ teaspoon sea salt

½ teaspoon ground cumin

¼ cup olive oil, plus more for drizzling

1 tablespoon filtered water (optional)

1. In a large pot that fits a steamer basket or insert, bring 1 inch of water to a boil. Add the lima beans and cover. Keep the water at a low boil. Cook for 15 minutes. This is longer than usual, so they're soft and easy to mash.

2. In a food processor or blender, combine the lima beans, pine nuts, lemon juice, dill, garlic, salt, and cumin. Puree the mixture until it's smooth.

3. With the blender running, slowly drizzle in the olive oil, 1 tablespoon at a time, blending to incorporate after each addition. If the hummus is dry, add water 1 teaspoon at a time until it reaches your desired consistency.

4. To serve, transfer to a serving dish and drizzle with additional olive oil to garnish. Store leftover hummus in an airtight container in the refrigerator for up to 7 days or in the freezer for up to 3 months.

TIP: A typical serving size is 2 tablespoons. I used ½ cup to get to 5 grams of fiber because this is a high-fiber snack whether you eat 2 tablespoons or ½ cup. Eating it with vegetables or crackers will add more fiber.

Per serving (½ cup): Calories: 346; Total fat: 27g; Total carbs: 22g; Cholesterol: 0mg; Fiber: 5g; Sugar: 0.5g; Protein: 7g; Sodium: 432mg

GREEN BEANS WITH GARLIC-GINGER SAUCE

Prep time: 5 minutes | **Cook time:** 10 minutes | **Makes** 6 servings

This is a quick and delicious recipe that's family friendly. Perfect for a weekday dinner, it goes well with a protein main dish and steamed rice. All you have to do is steam the beans and pour the sauce over them.

2 pounds green beans, trimmed

½ cup Garlic-Ginger Sauce (page 118)

¼ cup shelled sunflower seeds

1. In a medium pot that fits a steamer basket or insert, bring 1 inch of water to a boil. Add the green beans and cover. Steam for 3 to 5 minutes, depending on how crisp you like your beans.

2. To serve, pour the sauce over the top and sprinkle with sunflower seeds.

TIP: Instead of garlic-ginger sauce, you can use your favorite bottled sauce, peanut sauce, or coconut aminos, but keep in mind that the fiber will be slightly lower.

Per serving: Calories: 121; Total fat: 5.5g; Total carbs: 16g; Cholesterol: 0mg; Fiber: 5g; Sugar: 7.5g; Protein: 5g; Sodium: 379mg

FERMENTED JICAMA

Prep time: 10 minutes, plus 3 to 7 days to ferment | **Makes** 6 servings

The gut health benefits provided by fiber and probiotics make fermented vegetables a wise daily choice. If you're new to eating ferments, start with 2 tablespoons and increase slowly. You'll need a quart-size glass jar and a weight or small glass dish to keep things submerged. An airlock lid kit is recommended but not required (see Resources, page 130).

1½ tablespoons sea salt

2½ cups filtered water

1 medium jicama, peeled and cut into matchsticks

1 medium shallot, diced

1 tablespoon freshly squeezed lime juice

1. In a glass measuring cup, dissolve the salt in the water.

2. Pack the jicama and shallot into a glass jar, leaving 1 inch of headspace. Pour the lime juice and salt brine into the jar, covering the vegetables. Put a weight on top to completely submerge the vegetables so they don't mold.

3. If using an airlock lid, fill the chamber with water to the fill line and secure the chamber into the lid. Screw the lid onto the jar. Store the jar at 68°F to 77°F in a dark place for up to 7 days.

4. Taste the jicama daily on days 3 through 7, stopping when you like the taste. Jicama will get soft if it goes much longer than 7 days. Remove the airlock chamber from the jar and plug the hole with a stopper or switch to a plastic lid. Store in the refrigerator for up to 6 months.

> **TIP:** Avoid containers or lids with metal. The acidic ferment can corrode the metal and leach into your ferment if it touches the food.

Per serving (⅔ cup): Calories: 47; Total fat: 0g; Total carbs: 11g; Cholesterol: 0mg; Fiber: 5.5g; Sugar: 2.5g; Protein: 1g; Sodium: 180mg

SMOKY SPICED NUT AND SEED MIX

Prep time: 10 minutes | **Cook time:** 30 minutes | **Makes** 2 cups

Smoked paprika is derived from mild chile peppers that were dried over the smoke from an oak fire. The delicious flavor in this spice mix will probably remind you of barbecuing. Rather than the typical ¼-cup serving, I've used a more realistic ½-cup serving, which gives 5.5 grams of fiber and classifies it as a high-fiber snack.

2 tablespoons ghee, butter, or coconut oil

½ cup unsalted hazelnuts

½ cup unsalted almonds

½ cup unsalted pecans

½ cup raw pumpkin seeds (pepitas)

½ teaspoon sea salt

½ teaspoon smoked paprika

¼ teaspoon garlic powder

¼ teaspoon onion powder

1. Preheat the oven to 300°F. Line a baking sheet with parchment paper and set aside.

2. In a small saucepan, melt the ghee over low heat.

3. Meanwhile, in a medium bowl, toss the hazelnuts, almonds, pecans, and pumpkin seeds until mixed. Add the salt, paprika, garlic powder, and onion powder to the melted ghee and stir to combine. Pour the ghee over the nuts and toss to coat evenly.

4. Spread the nuts in a single layer on the baking sheet. Bake for 30 minutes, stirring every 10 minutes.

5. Spread the mixture out on paper towels to cool before serving. Store in an airtight container in a cool, dry place for up to 3 weeks. For longer-term storage, freeze the nuts on a parchment-lined baking sheet in a single layer just until they harden. Then transfer them to an airtight container in the freezer.

TIP: For variety, swap 1½ teaspoons of Tex-Mex Seasoning (page 121) for the salt and seasonings.

Per serving (½ cup): Calories: 442; Total fat: 42g; Total carbs: 10g; Cholesterol: 16mg; Fiber: 6g; Sugar: 2g; Protein: 12g; Sodium: 293mg

SESAME-CARROT-EDAMAME MEDLEY

Prep time: 10 minutes | **Cook time:** 10 minutes | **Makes** 4 servings

This is fast and easy to make and pairs well with the Asian-Inspired Turkey Loaf (page 71) and other chicken or fish dishes. It's also great in a lunch box because it's good eaten hot or cold. I used black sesame seeds for garnish because they still have their hulls, which contain calcium and other minerals. If black seeds aren't available, white will suffice.

4 medium carrots, cut into ⅛-inch-thick slices

8 ounces frozen shelled edamame (preferably organic)

2 tablespoons Garlic Oil (page 115) or olive oil plus 1 minced garlic clove

2 tablespoons orange juice

2 teaspoons sesame oil

2 teaspoons coconut aminos

2 medium scallions, green parts only, finely chopped

2 teaspoons untoasted black sesame seeds, for garnishing

1. In a large pot that fits a steamer basket or insert, bring 1 inch of water to a boil. Add the carrots. Cover and steam for 5 minutes. Add the edamame to the steamer basket and steam for 5 minutes longer, until the carrots are tender.

2. Meanwhile, in a small bowl, whisk together the garlic oil, orange juice, sesame oil, and coconut aminos.

3. Transfer the carrots and edamame to a serving bowl. Pour the oil mixture over the top and toss to evenly coat. Garnish with scallions and sesame seeds and serve. Store leftovers in an airtight container in the refrigerator for up to 5 days.

TIP: You can save a little time using frozen diced carrots instead of chopping fresh carrots. Just add them to the steamer basket with the edamame and steam for 5 minutes.

Per serving: Calories: 197; Total fat: 12g; Total carbs: 14g; Cholesterol: 0mg; Fiber: 6.5g; Sugar: 4.5g; Protein: 9g; Sodium: 102mg

ALMOND BUTTER CRACKERS

Prep time: 15 minutes | **Cook time:** 12 minutes | **Makes** 126 crackers

These crackers appeal to all ages—my grandsons devour them. These are best made with almond butter that has no added oil and will keep in an airtight container in the refrigerator for up to 7 days.

2 cups almond flour

⅓ cup coconut flour

⅓ cup psyllium husk powder

1 teaspoon sea salt, divided

½ cup pure creamy almond butter

½ cup filtered water

2 tablespoons raw local honey

1. Preheat the oven to 350°F. Cut 3 sheets of parchment paper to fit a baking sheet and set aside.

2. In a large bowl, mix the almond flour, coconut flour, psyllium, and ½ teaspoon of the salt, stirring until no lumps remain.

3. In a small bowl, whisk the almond butter, water, and honey until well combined. Combine the wet and dry ingredients in the large bowl and mix until a dough forms. Knead the dough for about 30 seconds, then separate it into 2 balls.

4. Roll each ball between 2 sheets of the parchment into a 1/16-inch-thick rectangle, about 11 × 14 inches. Reuse the top sheet for the second ball. Cut the dough in a grid of 9 columns and 7 rows into about 1½-inch squares with a knife or pizza cutter. Poke each cracker twice with a fork. Sprinkle with the remaining ½ teaspoon salt.

5. Transfer the crackers on the parchment to a baking sheet. Bake for 12 minutes, until golden brown. Cool before serving.

TIP: If you prefer, mix the dough in a food processor, mixing the wet ingredients first.

Per serving (14 crackers): Calories: 285; Total fat: 17g; Total carbs: 25g; Cholesterol: 0mg; Fiber: 10g; Sugar: 7.5g; Protein: 11g; Sodium: 261mg

PARSNIP-PEAR MASH

Prep time: 10 minutes | **Cook time:** 15 minutes | **Makes** 4 servings

This mash is a nice deviation from mashed potatoes. The pears help balance the sharp taste of parsnips and lower the glycemic load of the dish, while the mustard and herbs add to its flavor complexity. The vegetable broth can be reused and has a richly enhanced flavor that makes delicious soup.

3 large parsnips, peeled and cut into 1-inch pieces

2 medium pears, peeled, cored, and quartered lengthwise

4 cups vegetable broth

½ teaspoon sea salt

⅓ cup plain unsweetened goat or nondairy yogurt

2 tablespoons olive oil

1 tablespoon Dijon mustard

1½ teaspoons chopped fresh rosemary

1½ teaspoons fresh thyme leaves

¼ teaspoon ground black pepper

1. In a large saucepan, cover the parsnips and pears with the vegetable broth. Add the salt and bring to a boil over medium-high heat. Reduce the heat as necessary to continue boiling for about 15 minutes, or until the parsnips are completely fork-tender.

2. Drain and strain the broth into a quart-size jar or glass container with a lid. Refrigerate the broth for up to 5 days or freeze it for up to 3 months for use in other recipes.

3. Over low heat, using a hand mixer, immersion blender, or potato masher, mash the parsnips and pears with the yogurt and oil until smooth. Add the Dijon, rosemary, thyme, and pepper. Mix to incorporate.

4. Store leftovers in an airtight container in the refrigerator for up to 5 days or in the freezer for up to 3 months.

TIP: The protein in goat milk is different from that in cow milk, so some people can tolerate it. But if you can't, use coconut, almond, or cashew yogurt.

Per serving: Calories: 270; Total fat: 8g; Total carbs: 48g; Cholesterol: 4mg; Fiber: 12g; Sugar: 19g; Protein: 3g; Sodium: 949mg

THAI-INSPIRED FLATBREADS

Prep time: 10 minutes | **Cook time:** 15 minutes | **Makes** 4 servings

These delicious flatbreads are like a Thai-inspired pizza. They come together quickly when you have the sauce and flatbreads made ahead of time. Eat them as an appetizer, a snack, or a side dish. Add chicken to turn it into an entrée. If desired, garnish each flatbread after they come out of the oven with 1 to 2 teaspoons of cilantro or Thai basil and/or sprinkle with red pepper flakes.

4 flatbreads from Grain-Free Baguette, Rolls, or Flatbreads (page 124)

6 tablespoons Garlic-Ginger Sauce (page 118)

½ cup bean sprouts

1 large carrot, shredded

2 scallions, green parts only, chopped

½ cup dry-roasted peanuts, chopped

1. Preheat the oven to 400°F.

2. Place the flatbreads on a baking sheet or baking stone. Spread about 1½ tablespoons of sauce on each flatbread. In this order, top with about 2 tablespoons each of bean sprouts, carrot, scallions, and peanuts.

3. Bake for 15 minutes. Serve immediately or store in an airtight container in the refrigerator for up to 5 days, including the time since the bread and sauce were made.

> **TIP:** You won't get as much fiber, but you can use a small gluten-free pizza crust and teriyaki sauce if you don't have the flatbreads or garlic-ginger sauce made.

Per serving (1 flatbread): Calories: 462; Total fat: 25g; Total carbs: 44g; Cholesterol: 0mg; Fiber: 16g; Sugar: 9g; Protein: 17g; Sodium: 839mg

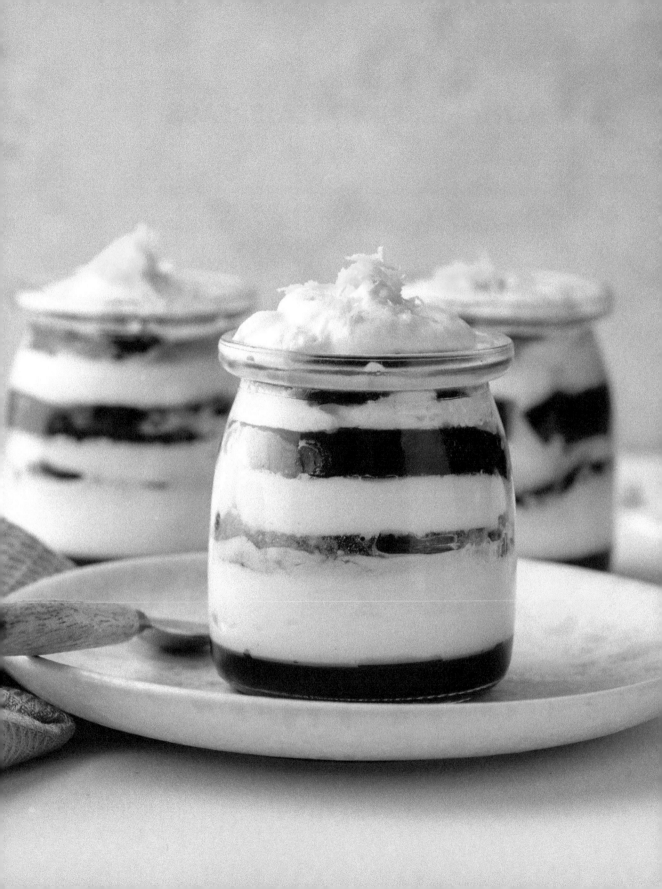

Chapter 6

DESSERTS

CRANBERRY GELATIN

Prep time: 10 minutes, plus 2 hours to chill | **Cook time:** 5 minutes
Makes 3 servings

This is such a versatile recipe. If you don't like cranberry juice, you can use your favorite juice instead, as long as it contains no pulp, during the Clear Liquid Phase. You can also add chunks of fruit after that phase.

3 cups unsweetened cranberry juice, divided

2 tablespoons unflavored gelatin, preferably grass-fed

1 tablespoon raw local honey (optional)

¼ teaspoon Himalayan pink salt

1. In a bowl, combine 1½ cups of the juice with the gelatin. Allow it to sit for 1 minute.

2. In the meantime, in a small saucepan, gently heat the remaining 1½ cups of juice over medium-high heat until steam rises from the top. Turn off the heat and add the cold juice-gelatin mixture. Stir well until the gelatin is dissolved. Add the honey (if using) and salt and stir until it is incorporated.

3. Pour the gelatin mixture into an 8-inch square glass dish. Cover it with a lid or plastic wrap and allow it to cool completely in the refrigerator for 2 hours.

4. Cut into squares, desired shapes, or just scoop into bowls. Store in the refrigerator, covered, for up to 7 days.

TIP: In the High-Fiber Phase, add 1 (8-ounce) can of crushed pineapple (drained), 1 (11-ounce) can of mandarin oranges (drained), and 3 tablespoons of chopped pecans for a chunky dessert salad.

Per serving: Calories: 122; Total fat: 0.5g; Total carbs: 32g; Cholesterol: 0mg; Fiber: 0g; Sugar: 32g; Protein: 1g; Sodium: 206mg

KOMBUCHA GELATIN

Prep time: 5 minutes, plus 2 hours 10 minutes to chill
Cook time: 5 minutes | **Makes** 2 servings

Kombucha is a fermented tea beverage with antioxidants and gut-healthy probiotics. You can use your favorite kombucha to flavor this fast, easy gelatin. I chose ginger because it contains gingerol, a potent compound with antioxidant and anti-inflammatory properties that can help alleviate nausea, constipation, and bloating. Kombucha brands I like include GT's, Brew Dr. Kombucha, and Live.

½ cup filtered water

1 tablespoon unflavored gelatin, preferably grass-fed

12 ounces ginger kombucha

1. In a small saucepan, bring the water to a boil over high heat. Remove the pan from the heat and stir in the gelatin until it is completely dissolved. Let the mixture cool to room temperature for about 10 minutes before combining with the kombucha so you don't kill the probiotics in the kombucha.

2. Add the kombucha and pour into serving dishes or storage containers. Refrigerate for 2 hours, or until the gelatin is set. Store in an airtight container in the refrigerator for up to 7 days. Freezing can kill the probiotics.

TIP: In the High-Fiber Phase, you can use a kombucha with chia seeds, if desired, or add 1 to 2 tablespoons of chia seeds.

Per serving: Calories: 42; Total fat: 0g; Total carbs: 8g; Cholesterol: 0mg; Fiber: 0g; Sugar: 7.5g; Protein: 0g; Sodium: 5mg

PEACH UPSIDE-DOWN CAKE

Prep time: 15 minutes | **Cook time:** 40 minutes | **Makes** 8 servings

This cake was created as a special low-fiber treat for your recovery. Although it's a reduced-sugar recipe using coconut sugar and honey rather than refined white or brown sugar and a low-fiber rice flour mix to aid your recovery, there's nothing bland about this sweet delight.

1 (15-ounce) can juice-packed peach halves

2 tablespoons ghee, butter, or coconut oil

⅓ cup coconut sugar

¼ cup coconut oil

¼ cup honey

1 large egg

1 teaspoon pure vanilla extract

1 teaspoon baking powder

½ teaspoon baking soda

¼ teaspoon sea salt

1 cup Low-Fiber Flour Blend (page 119)

1 cup coconut cream

1. Preheat the oven to 350°F.

2. Drain the juice from the can of peaches into a glass measuring cup and set aside.

3. Melt the ghee in an 8-inch square or round pan in the oven. Remove the pan from the oven and stir in the coconut sugar and 1 tablespoon of the reserved juice. Spread the mixture out evenly in the bottom of the pan. Cut each peach half into 4 slices and arrange them on top of the ghee mixture.

4. In a medium mixing bowl, cream the coconut oil and honey with a hand mixer on medium for 1 to 2 minutes, until the mixture is slightly fluffy. Add the egg and vanilla and beat for 2 minutes. Add the baking powder, baking soda, and salt and mix well. Mix in ½ cup of the reserved juice from the peaches. Gradually add the flour and beat for about 2 minutes.

5. Spread the cake batter over the peaches and bake for about 40 minutes, or until the cake springs back when you gently press on the center with a finger. Cool for 5 minutes, then invert the pan onto a plate. Note that dark caramelization does not mean burned. Cut into 8 rectangles or wedges (depending on the shape of your pan).

6. Serve warm, drizzled with the coconut cream. Cover and store leftovers in an airtight container in the refrigerator for up to 5 days or in the freezer for up to 3 months.

TIP: You can buy peach slices in juice, but the slices are a little thick for a topping.

Per serving (1 piece): Calories: 312; Total fat: 16g; Total carbs: 38g; Cholesterol: 31mg; Fiber: 1g; Sugar: 20g; Protein: 1g; Sodium: 100mg

HIBISCUS-POMEGRANATE YOGURT PARFAIT

Prep time: 15 minutes, plus 2 hours to set | **Cook time:** 5 minutes
Makes 6 servings

The coconut yogurt in this parfait adds a rich creaminess. You'll need 6 (6-ounce) glass dishes so you can see the beautiful layers in this dessert. I use yogurt jars because they have screw-on tops, making them easy to refrigerate and store.

1½ cups filtered water

¼ cup unflavored gelatin, preferably grass-fed, divided

½ cup dried hibiscus flowers

2 cups unsweetened coconut yogurt

2 tablespoons raw local honey

1 teaspoon ground ginger

1 cup unsweetened pomegranate juice

1 tablespoon finely grated lemon zest

1. In a small saucepan, bring the water to a boil over high heat. Remove the pan from the heat and stir in 2 tablespoons of the gelatin until it dissolves. Add the hibiscus flowers and steep for 10 minutes.

2. In a medium bowl, whisk the yogurt with the remaining 2 tablespoons of gelatin, the honey, and the ginger to mix thoroughly. Cover and refrigerate.

3. Strain the hibiscus tea into a 2-cup glass measuring cup or bowl. Discard the flowers. Add the pomegranate juice and stir.

4. Pour some tea mixture into each jar or dish to make a layer about ⅝ inch thick. Pour the remaining liquid into an 8 x 8-inch pan or dish. Put the jars and pan in the refrigerator for 2 hours, or until the gelatin is set.

5. Spoon enough yogurt into each jar to make another equivalent-size layer. Using a glass, cookie cutter, or dull knife, cut circles out of the gelatin in the pan to fit inside the jars. Using a spatula, gently lift the circles from the pan. Fold them in half and insert them into the jar on top of the yogurt. You can add the extra gelatin that didn't make it in the circle or eat it separately. Top the gelatin with another layer of yogurt and sprinkle with the lemon zest.

6. Store in airtight containers in the refrigerator for up to 5 days.

TIP: You can find hibiscus at Mexican markets or online (see Resources, page 130), or use 6 hibiscus tea bags. If you want a little tang, swap goat milk yogurt or Greek-style yogurt for the coconut yogurt.

Per serving (1 parfait): Calories: 106; Total fat: 3g; Total carbs: 22g; Cholesterol: 0mg; Fiber: 2g; Sugar: 18g; Protein: 0g; Sodium: 13mg

QUICK TAPIOCA PUDDING

Prep time: 5 minutes, plus 20 minutes to cool | **Cook time:** 20 minutes
Makes 4 servings

Who doesn't love the sweet, creamy-yet-sticky texture of tapioca pudding? With instant tapioca such as Minute Tapioca, this pudding cooks quickly to satiate your sweet tooth and tastes better than premade pudding.

2¼ cups plain unsweetened almond milk

3 tablespoons plus ¾ teaspoon egg whites

1½ tablespoons arrowroot starch/flour

1½ tablespoons filtered water

2½ tablespoons instant granulated tapioca

¼ cup raw local honey

¾ teaspoon pure vanilla extract

Pinch ground nutmeg

1. In a medium saucepan, bring the milk to a boil over medium-high heat. Be careful not to scorch it.

2. Meanwhile, in a medium mixing bowl with a mixer on high speed, beat the egg whites until they are fluffy. Set aside.

3. In a small bowl or cup, whisk the arrowroot and water. Set aside.

4. Add the tapioca to the boiling milk. Reduce the heat to medium. Cook, stirring often, for about 10 minutes, until the tapioca is completely transparent. Add the arrowroot mixture and stir as the mixture boils for another minute.

5. Remove the pan from the heat. Stir in the honey, vanilla, and nutmeg until blended. Fold in the beaten egg whites.

6. Cool for 20 minutes, then stir before serving or refrigerating in an airtight container for up to 1 week or freezing for up to 3 months.

TIP: If you don't have a mixer, beat the egg whites by hand for 15 to 20 minutes or pulse in a blender.

Per serving: Calories: 120; Total fat: 1.5g; Total carbs: 24g; Cholesterol: 0mg; Fiber: 0g; Sugar: 17g; Protein: 2g; Sodium: 126mg

RASPBERRY NICE CREAM

Prep time: 10 minutes, plus overnight to soak | **Makes** 4 servings

Who needs an ice-cream maker? A high-speed blender is all that's needed to make this "nice cream" both quickly and easily. Made with whole food ingredients, this raw vegan dessert is much healthier than ice cream.

½ cup cashews, soaked overnight and drained

2 medium frozen bananas

3 cups frozen raspberries

1. In a high-speed blender, blend the cashews until they are nearly smooth. Add the bananas and raspberries and blend on high until smooth.

2. This should be the consistency of soft-serve ice cream and is best served immediately, but it can be stored in the freezer for up to 3 months. Remove the nice cream from the freezer about 20 minutes before you want to eat it.

> **TIP:** A dollop of chilled or whipped coconut milk and a sprinkling of 1 tablespoon each of unsweetened, shredded coconut and finely chopped nuts turns nice cream into a fancy dessert.

Per serving: Calories: 162; Total fat: 6g; Total carbs: 26g; Cholesterol: 0mg; Fiber: 5g; Sugar: 11g; Protein: 4g; Sodium: 3mg

MACADAMIA-COCONUT BAR COOKIES

Prep time: 10 minutes, plus 30 minutes to cool | **Cook time:** 40 minutes
Makes 8 bars

Macadamia nuts and coconut are a perfect combination for both flavor and fiber content. The navy beans add even more fiber, a smooth texture, and moisture. Applesauce also adds moisture. You'll be transferring the batter ingredients back and forth from the blender to the mixing bowl, so don't clean up until the batter is in the pan.

¼ cup coconut oil, plus more for greasing

½ cup gluten-free rolled oats

½ cup coconut sugar

½ teaspoon baking soda

½ teaspoon baking powder

¼ teaspoon sea salt

2 large eggs

½ cup (3.9-ounce container) unsweetened applesauce

2 teaspoons pure vanilla extract

1 (15-ounce) can navy or great northern beans, drained and rinsed

½ cup macadamia nuts, roughly chopped

½ cup unsweetened shredded coconut

1. Preheat the oven to 350°F. Grease an 8-inch square glass pan with oil and set aside.

2. If the coconut oil is solid, melt it in a small saucepan over low heat or in the microwave for about 15 seconds.

3. Place the oats in a blender and blend on medium until powdery. Add the coconut sugar, baking soda, baking powder, and salt. Pulse a few times, just enough to mix the ingredients and eliminate any lumps in the coconut sugar.

4. In a medium bowl, beat the eggs. Stir in the applesauce and vanilla. Add the oil and whisk well. Add the dry ingredients from the blender and stir to combine and form the batter.

5. In the blender, process the beans and about 1 cup of the batter on high speed until the beans are completely mashed; add the remaining batter and blend for about 30 seconds.

6. Transfer the batter back to the bowl and fold in the nuts and coconut. Spread the batter evenly in the prepared pan and bake for about 40 minutes, or until the top cracks slightly and the edges pull away from the sides of the pan. A toothpick will come out clean before this happens, but it may still be gooey, so don't rush it.

7. Cool for 30 minutes before cutting into 8 bars and serving. Store any leftover bars in an airtight container in the refrigerator for up to 7 days or in the freezer for up to 3 months.

TIP: Chopping round nuts can be tricky. You can use the flat side of a large knife or a cleaver to crush them or use a food processor or chopper. You can also use a different nut and/or add cacao nibs or chocolate chips, if tolerated.

Per serving (1 bar): Calories: 328; Total fat: 19g; Total carbs: 30g; Cholesterol: 46mg; Fiber: 5.5g; Sugar: 12g; Protein: 7g; Sodium: 295mg

APPLE CRUMBLE

Prep time: 15 minutes | **Cook time:** 45 minutes | **Makes** 6 servings

Apple crumble is a classic that works as well for dessert as it does for breakfast. This crumble captures the flavors of tender baked apples, cinnamon, and a buttery coconut sugar topping. It's comfort food made healthier!

5 medium Granny Smith apples, cored and sliced

3 tablespoons plain unsweetened almond milk

½ teaspoon ground cinnamon

¾ cup gluten-free rolled oats

½ cup coconut sugar

½ cup chopped walnuts

¼ cup cold ghee, butter, or coconut oil

1. Preheat the oven to 375°F.

2. Spread the apple slices evenly in a 9 x 9-inch baking dish. Drizzle the milk over them and sprinkle with cinnamon.

3. In a medium bowl, mix the oats, sugar, and walnuts. Using a fork or pastry blender, cut in the ghee until crumbly. Don't overdo it, or you'll have a pasty mixture.

4. Sprinkle the oat mixture over the apples. Bake for 45 minutes, or until the apples are soft. If the crumble mixture starts to burn, cover the dish with aluminum foil.

TIP: I use an apple corer/slicer and then slice the slices in half lengthwise so they're thinner and bake more quickly. You can substitute fresh peaches or pears for the apples, if desired.

Per serving: Calories: 320; Total fat: 16g; Total carbs: 43g; Cholesterol: 22mg; Fiber: 6g; Sugar: 29g; Protein: 3g; Sodium: 24mg

CHIA-MANGO PARFAIT

Prep time: 10 minutes, plus 3 hours to chill | **Makes** 4 servings

This is a super easy and delicious dessert that requires only 10 minutes of prep time and can be made in advance for meal prepping or guests. For meal prepping, I like to use 6-ounce yogurt jars. For guests, it's pretty in parfait dishes topped with a dollop of chilled or whipped coconut cream.

1⅔ cups full-fat coconut milk or another nut milk

6 tablespoons chia seeds

1 tablespoon raw local honey

1 teaspoon pure vanilla extract

1 large mango, peeled and roughly chopped

1. In medium bowl, combine the coconut milk, chia seeds, honey, and vanilla. Mix well and pour into dessert dishes or jars. Refrigerate for at least 3 hours.

2. In a blender, puree the mango on high. Remove the pudding from the refrigerator. Give it a stir, then top it with the mango puree.

3. Serve immediately or store in the refrigerator in airtight containers for up to 5 days.

TIP: If you prefer a smooth pudding, blend the milk–chia seed mixture in a blender until smooth before refrigerating. If necessary, sub the fresh mango with 1 cup of frozen chunks, thawed. You may need to add 1 or 2 teaspoons of water for pureeing.

Per serving: Calories: 333; Total fat: 25g; Total carbs: 27g; Cholesterol: 0mg; Fiber: 8g; Sugar: 17g; Protein: 5g; Sodium: 16mg

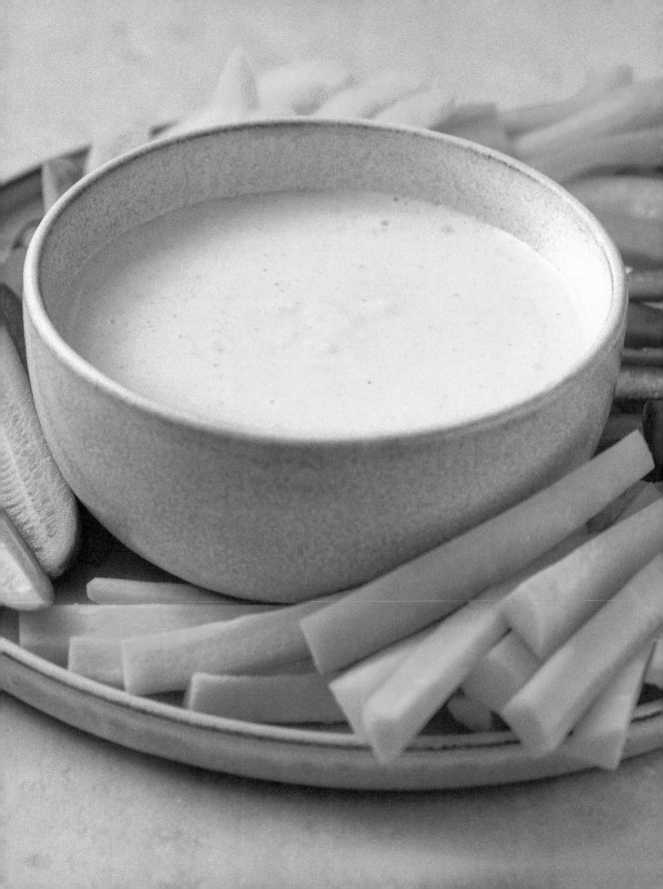

Chapter 7

STAPLES

CHICKEN BONE BROTH

Prep time: 15 minutes | **Cook time:** 24 hours | **Makes** 16 cups

Slow cooking bones with an acid like vinegar leaches nutrients such as collagen and amino acids from the bones into the broth. The amino acids glutamine and glycine can help heal the intestines, reduce inflammation, and protect against leaky gut. This flavorful broth uses low-FODMAP vegetables.

Bones from 2 pasture-raised chickens

16 cups filtered water

2 large leeks, green parts only, roughly chopped

2 medium carrots, roughly chopped

½ medium celeriac, roughly chopped

¼ cup raw apple cider vinegar

1 medium bay leaf

1 teaspoon poultry seasoning

1 teaspoon sea salt

½ teaspoon ground black pepper (optional)

1. If you're using bones that haven't been previously cooked, roast them at 425°F for about 30 minutes on a parchment-lined baking sheet.

2. In a large pot, combine the bones, water, leeks, carrots, celeriac, vinegar, bay leaf, poultry seasoning, salt, and pepper (if using), submerging the bones in the water. Bring to a boil over medium-high heat. Reduce the heat to low and simmer for 16 to 24 hours, until the bones are soft. Keep the simmer gentle so the broth stays clear. Skim off any foam, adding water as needed to keep the bones submerged.

3. Strain the broth through a cheesecloth-lined mesh strainer after cooling. Use the broth immediately or store it in an airtight container in the refrigerator for 3 days or in the freezer for up to 3 months.

TIP: You can cook this in 90 minutes using an Instant Pot or pressure cooker. To make beef broth, use bones from grass-fed and -finished cattle and omit the poultry seasoning.

Per serving (1 cup): Calories: 41; Total fat: 0g; Total carbs: 0g; Cholesterol: 5mg; Fiber: 0g; Sugar: 0g; Protein: 9g; Sodium: 303mg

LOW-FIBER

GARLIC OIL

Prep time: 5 minutes, plus 45 minutes to cool | **Cook time:** 5 minutes
Makes 1 cup

This is a fast, easy, and inexpensive way to have delicious, low-FODMAP garlic oil. FODMAPs are not fat-soluble, so you can cook the garlic in the oil and then strain it out along with the FODMAPs. This method does not produce a shelf-stable oil. For that, you need to acidify and infuse the oil (see Resources, page 130) or buy a ready-made garlic-infused oil.

1 garlic head, separated into cloves

1 cup olive oil

1. Smash the garlic cloves with the back of a chef's knife to loosen the peels and crush them slightly. Discard the peels.

2. In a small saucepan, bring the garlic and olive oil to a simmer over medium heat. Do not boil it, or the oil will be damaged and the flavor will be off. Reduce the heat to low and cook for 3 to 5 minutes, until the garlic is lightly brown and slightly crisp. Watch carefully so it doesn't burn.

3. Remove the pan from the heat and let it cool for 30 to 45 minutes to infuse more flavor. Strain the oil into a jar or airtight container.

4. Store the oil in the refrigerator for up to 5 days or freeze for up to 1 year. Do not store at room temperature. If you need the oil runny to drizzle or for salad dressing, take it out of the refrigerator at least 30 minutes in advance.

TIP: If you want a stronger garlic flavor, leave the garlic in the oil and strain it when you use it.

Per serving (1 tablespoon): Calories: 119; Total fat: 13g; Total carbs: 0g; Cholesterol: 0mg; Fiber: 0g; Sugar: 0g; Protein: 0g; Sodium: 4mg

BREAKFAST SAUSAGE SEASONING

Prep time: 5 minutes | **Makes** about ¼ cup

This is the closest I could come to the flavor of the Southern sausage my grandmother used to make. Many commercial sausages contain unhealthy sugars, MSG, corn syrup, and flavorings. This mix allows you to use only wholesome ingredients and choose the type and quality of protein you want to use. The maple sugar can be omitted or substituted with 1 tablespoon of coconut sugar. Alternatively, you could add 1 tablespoon of maple syrup when seasoning the meat. This recipe will season 2 pounds of meat.

1 tablespoon maple sugar

1 tablespoon dried parsley

2 teaspoons sea salt

2 teaspoons rubbed sage

1 teaspoon paprika

1 teaspoon ground black pepper

½ teaspoon dried marjoram

¼ teaspoon dried thyme

1. In a spice mill or coffee grinder, grind the maple sugar, parsley, salt, sage, paprika, pepper, marjoram, and thyme until the herbs are evenly dispersed with no large leaves remaining. Alternatively, you can use a mortar and pestle or the back of a spoon in a bowl.

2. Store the seasoning in an airtight container for up to 1 year.

TIP: To make sausage patties, sprinkle 1½ tablespoons of seasoning over 1 pound of ground meat. Mix thoroughly, and then form the meat into ¼-pound patties. To store uncooked patties, put parchment paper between them and refrigerate for up to 5 days or freeze for up to 3 months in an airtight container. To cook, preheat the oven to 400°F. Place the patties on a baking sheet lined with parchment paper. Bake for 10 minutes, flip, and bake another 5 to 10 minutes until cooked through. Let them cool, then refrigerate in an airtight container for up to 4 days or freeze for up to 3 months.

Per serving (1 teaspoon): Calories: 4; Total fat: 0g; Total carbs: 1g; Cholesterol: 0mg; Fiber: 0g; Sugar: 0.5g; Protein: 0g; Sodium: 388mg

TENDER STEWED CHICKEN

Prep time: 15 minutes, plus up to 24 hours to marinate
Cook time: 40 minutes | **Makes** 6 servings

I make this recipe as is for freezing, but for specific dishes, you can add complementary herbs and spices to the pot. Save the bones to make bone broth, and cool and strain the broth into an airtight container for use in other recipes. Freeze both for up to 3 months.

⅔ cup raw local honey

⅓ cup sea salt

2 tablespoons ground black pepper

1 (5½-pound) whole chicken, roughly chopped

4 cups Chicken Bone Broth (page 114)

2 cups filtered water

1. Place the honey, salt, and pepper in a gallon zip-top bag and mix well. Add the chicken and massage until thoroughly coated. Refrigerate for 8 to 24 hours.

2. Rinse the chicken well and put it in a bowl of ice water for 1 hour to remove more salt.

3. Drain the chicken and layer the pieces in a large Dutch oven with the smaller pieces on top. Add the broth and enough water to submerge the chicken. Cover and bring to a boil over medium-high heat. Keep it at a low boil for 40 minutes, or until the thickest chicken piece reaches an internal temperature of 165°F.

4. Transfer the chicken to a platter to cool for 15 minutes, or until it is cool enough to handle, reserving the broth. Debone and slice, shred, or cube the chicken. Refrigerate the chicken in an airtight container for 3 to 4 days or freeze for up to 3 months.

TIP: You can skip the marinating and soaking in this recipe, but I recommend it if time permits.

Per serving (½ cup shredded): Calories: 290; Total fat: 11g; Total carbs: 1g; Cholesterol: 134mg; Fiber: 0g; Sugar: 1g; Protein: 44g; Sodium: 299mg

GARLIC-GINGER SAUCE

Prep time: 5 minutes | **Makes** ½ cup

Garlic and ginger will give your dish a delicious Asian flair. Serve the sauce over fish, poultry, or veggies in dishes like Salmon and Green Peas with Garlic-Ginger Sauce (page 69) or Green Beans with Garlic-Ginger Sauce (page 91).

⅓ cup coconut aminos

2 tablespoons roasted tahini

2 tablespoons orange juice

1 large garlic clove, peeled

1 (⅓-inch) piece fresh ginger root, peeled

1. In a small food processor or blender, blend the coconut aminos, tahini, orange juice, garlic, and ginger until the garlic and ginger pieces are tiny or not visible.

2. Store leftovers in an airtight container in the refrigerator for up to 5 days or in the freezer for up to 3 months.

> **TIP:** You can swap the coconut aminos for gluten-free low-sodium tamari if you prefer a saltier sauce.

Per serving (1 tablespoon): Calories: 34; Total fat: 2g; Total carbs: 3g; Cholesterol: 0mg; Fiber: 0g; Sugar: 2g; Protein: 1g; Sodium: 277mg

LOW-FIBER FLOUR BLEND

Prep time: 5 minutes | **Makes** 4 cups

Most gluten-free flour mixes contain whole-grain flours like sorghum and brown rice, which aren't allowed in the Low-Fiber Phase of the diverticulitis diet. Therefore, I came up with a blend using white rice and some necessary starches and binders specifically for this phase.

2 cups white rice flour

1 cup tapioca starch/ flour

1 cup cornstarch or potato starch

2 teaspoons xanthan gum

1. In a gallon zip-top bag, mix the rice flour, tapioca starch, cornstarch, and xanthan gum until thoroughly mixed.

2. Store at room temperature, out of direct light, for up to 6 months or in the freezer for up to 1 year.

TIP: When using this flour, don't expect foods to rise or brown in the same way they do with wheat flour, and expect a bit longer cooking time.

Per serving (¼ cup): Calories: 131; Total fat: 0g; Total carbs: 30g; Cholesterol: 0mg; Fiber: 0.5g; Sugar: 0g; Protein: 1g; Sodium: 15mg

HERBED RICE FLOUR BISCUITS

Prep time: 15 minutes | **Cook time:** 15 minutes | **Makes** 6 servings

If you have a bread craving, these biscuits will satisfy it. If you don't, you will when you smell these baking.

⅓ cup plain unsweetened almond milk

1 teaspoon raw apple cider vinegar

1 cup Low-Fiber Flour Blend (page 119) for drop biscuits; plus 3 tablespoons for rolled biscuits

1 teaspoon baking powder

1 teaspoon cream of tartar

1 teaspoon dried dill weed

½ teaspoon sea salt

¼ teaspoon baking soda

3 tablespoons cold ghee, butter, or coconut oil

1 large egg

1. Preheat the oven to 375°F.

2. In a small bowl, mix the milk and vinegar. Set aside for 5 minutes.

3. Meanwhile, in a large bowl, combine the flour, baking powder, cream of tartar, dill weed, salt, and baking soda. Stir to mix well. With a pastry blender or fork, cut the ghee into the flour mixture until the particles are fine.

4. Whisk the egg into the milk mixture then pour into the large bowl and mix well.

5. For drop biscuits: Drop 6 large spoonfuls of dough onto an ungreased baking sheet. For rolled biscuits: Dust the surface with flour and knead the dough for 30 seconds. Roll it out ½ inch thick between 2 sheets of parchment paper. Using a biscuit cutter, donut cutter, or a glass, cut the dough into circles, rerolling as necessary. Arrange on an ungreased baking sheet. Bake for 13 to 15 minutes, until firm.

6. Refrigerate cooled biscuits in an airtight container for 7 to 10 days, or freeze for up to 12 months.

TIP: The dill can be swapped for other herbs, such as dried parsley, basil, sage, thyme, or rosemary.

Per serving (1 biscuit): Calories: 160; Total fat: 7.5g; Total carbs: 21g; Cholesterol: 47mg; Fiber: 0.5g; Sugar: 0g; Protein: 2g; Sodium: 279mg

TEX-MEX SEASONING

Prep time: 5 minutes | **Makes** about ⅔ cup

Store-bought seasoning often contains gluten and other additives, and the flavor can't compare with this homemade version. This seasoning uses only wholesome ingredients and is great for more than ground beef and turkey taco meat. Try sprinkling it on chicken, fish, and veggies, or use it in Tex-Mex Flatbreads (page 83). This makes enough to season about 4½ pounds of meat.

¼ cup chili powder

4 teaspoons arrowroot starch/flour

1 tablespoon ground cumin

1 tablespoon onion powder

1 tablespoon paprika

2 teaspoons garlic powder

2 teaspoons sea salt

1 teaspoon dried Mexican oregano

1 teaspoon ground black pepper

1. In a small bowl or jar, combine the chili powder, arrowroot, cumin, onion powder, paprika, garlic powder, salt, oregano, and pepper until thoroughly combined.

2. For 1 pound of meat, use 7 teaspoons of seasoning and ¼ cup water. Store unused seasoning in an airtight container for up to 1 year.

> **TIP:** You can control the heat by using mild or hot chili powder and/or adding red pepper flakes or cayenne pepper.

Per serving (2 teaspoons): Calories: 9; Total fat: 0g; Total carbs: 5g; Cholesterol: 0mg; Fiber: 0.5g; Sugar: 0g; Protein: 0g; Sodium: 292mg

SAVORY SAUCE AND DIP

Prep time: 10 minutes, plus 8 hours to soak | **Makes** 2¾ cups

This tasty sauce/dip is extremely versatile. Use it when you want an extra flavor punch as a sauce for veggies, rice, or bowls; a spread on sandwiches or burgers; a dip for chips, raw veggies, or Rice Flour Crackers (page 89); or a flavor and fiber booster in soup.

½ cup raw almonds, soaked overnight and drained

½ cup olive oil

½ (15-ounce) can navy beans, drained and rinsed

1 tablespoon nutritional yeast

1 large garlic clove, peeled

1 teaspoon raw apple cider vinegar

¾ teaspoon sea salt

½ teaspoon curry powder

½ cup filtered water

1. In a high-speed blender, combine the almonds, olive oil, navy beans, nutritional yeast, garlic, vinegar, salt, and curry powder and blend on high until smooth. Add as much of the water as desired to reach a sauce or dip consistency.

2. Serve or store in an airtight container the refrigerator for up to 4 days.

TIP: With the oil, this will solidify when refrigerated, so take it out of the refrigerator at least 30 minutes in advance; you can also warm it for about 10 seconds in the microwave or in a saucepan over low heat for about 2 minutes. Freeze or eat the leftover beans.

Per serving (1 tablespoon): Calories: 37; Total fat: 3g; Total carbs: 1g; Cholesterol: 0mg; Fiber: 0.5g; Sugar: 0g; Protein: 1g; Sodium: 55mg

SALSA VERDE

Prep time: 15 minutes | **Cook time:** 15 minutes | **Makes** 3 to 4 cups

Hopefully, you've recovered and can enjoy the ingredients in this delicious salsa. This sauce is mild, but you can add more jalapeño if you tolerate it. It's great as an enchilada sauce or salsa. Check it out on Chicken Enchiladas (page 73) and Tex-Mex Flatbreads (page 83).

12 large tomatillos, halved lengthwise

2 large poblano peppers, halved lengthwise and seeded

1 large jalapeño pepper, halved lengthwise and seeded

1 large white onion, cut lengthwise into quarters

4 large garlic cloves, peeled

1½ teaspoons sea salt, divided

1 cup chopped fresh cilantro

2 tablespoons freshly squeezed lime juice

1. Preheat the oven to 425°F.

2. On a large baking sheet, arrange the tomatillos, poblano and jalapeño peppers, onion, and garlic, cut-sides up. Sprinkle with about ½ teaspoon of the salt. Roast for 12 to 15 minutes. Watch carefully and remove the baking sheet from the oven as soon as any of the vegetables start to char.

3. In a food processor or blender, pulse the cilantro and lime juice until roughly chopped. Add the roasted vegetables from the tray to the blender and process until it reaches your desired consistency. Taste and add up to the remaining 1 teaspoon of salt, as desired.

4. Use immediately or store in an airtight container in the refrigerator for up to 5 days or in the freezer for up to 3 months.

TIP: Consider using this pureed as a sauce on grilled or cooked chicken or fish, chunky in a taco bowl or rice, or served cold like traditional salsa.

Per serving (⅓ cup): Calories: 47; Total fat: 1g; Total carbs: 10g; Cholesterol: 0mg; Fiber: 2.5g; Sugar: 5g; Protein: 1g; Sodium: 663mg

GRAIN-FREE BAGUETTE, ROLLS, OR FLATBREADS

Prep time: 15 minutes | **Cook time:** 35 minutes to 1 hour | **Makes** 6 servings

Somehow the smell of fresh baked bread takes us back to childhood. This guilt-free bread is low-carb and high-fiber.

1¾ cups almond flour

⅓ cup coconut flour

⅓ cup psyllium husk powder

¼ cup tapioca starch/ flour

3 tablespoons ground flaxseed

1 teaspoon baking soda

½ teaspoon sea salt

1⅓ cups filtered water

2 tablespoons raw apple cider vinegar

1. Preheat the oven to 375°F. Line a large baking sheet with parchment paper and set aside.

2. In a large bowl, combine the almond flour, coconut flour, psyllium, tapioca starch, flaxseed, baking soda, and salt. Mix to remove lumps.

3. Add the water and vinegar to the bowl and mix until the dry ingredients are completely wet. Let the mixture sit for about 1 minute.

4. Knead the dough for about 1 minute, until it becomes tight and smooth. Shape the dough into 1 loaf, 2 baguette, 10 dinner rolls, or 6 (7-inch-diameter) flatbreads and place them on the baking sheet. Allow space between them for rising and browning on all sides.

5. Bake the loaf for 1 hour, the baguette for 40 minutes, or the rolls and flatbreads for 35 minutes, until the centers are firm when pressed with your fingertip.

6. Store in an airtight container in the refrigerator for 7 to 10 days, or freeze for up to 12 months.

TIP: For the High-Fiber Phase meal plan (page 25), make 4 rolls and 2 flatbreads.

Per serving: Calories: 290; Total fat: 13g; Total carbs: 32g; Cholesterol: 0mg; Fiber: 13g; Sugar: 3.5g; Protein: 11g; Sodium: 408mg

MEASUREMENT CONVERSIONS

VOLUME EQUIVALENTS	U.S. STANDARD	U.S. STANDARD (OUNCES)	METRIC (APPROXIMATE)
LIQUID	2 tablespoons	1 fl. oz.	30 mL
	¼ cup	2 fl. oz.	60 mL
	½ cup	4 fl. oz.	120 mL
	1 cup	8 fl. oz.	240 mL
	1½ cups	12 fl. oz.	355 mL
	2 cups or 1 pint	16 fl. oz.	475 mL
	4 cups or 1 quart	32 fl. oz.	1 L
	1 gallon	128 fl. oz.	4 L
DRY	⅛ teaspoon	–	0.5 mL
	¼ teaspoon	–	1 mL
	½ teaspoon	–	2 mL
	¾ teaspoon	–	4 mL
	1 teaspoon	–	5 mL
	1 tablespoon	–	15 mL
	¼ cup	–	59 mL
	⅓ cup	–	79 mL
	½ cup	–	118 mL
	⅔ cup	–	156 mL
	¾ cup	–	177 mL
	1 cup	–	235 mL
	2 cups or 1 pint	–	475 mL
	3 cups	–	700 mL
	4 cups or 1 quart	–	1 L
	½ gallon	–	2 L
	1 gallon	–	4 L

OVEN TEMPERATURES

FAHRENHEIT	CELSIUS (APPROXIMATE)
250°F	120°C
300°F	150°C
325°F	165°C
350°F	180°C
375°F	190°C
400°F	200°C
425°F	220°C
450°F	230°C

WEIGHT EQUIVALENTS

U.S. STANDARD	METRIC (APPROXIMATE)
½ ounce	15 g
1 ounce	30 g
2 ounces	60 g
4 ounces	115 g
8 ounces	225 g
12 ounces	340 g
16 ounces or 1 pound	455 g

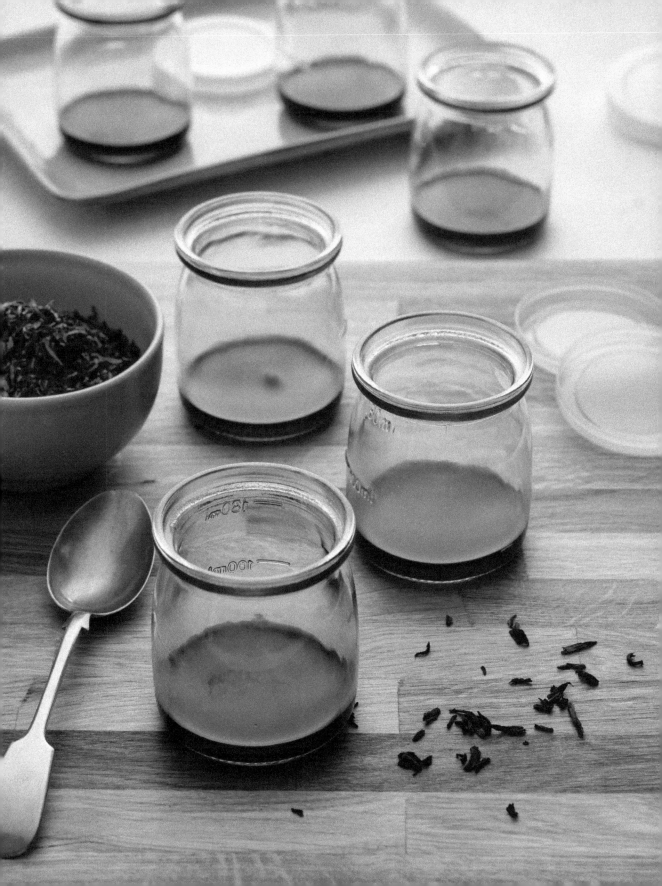

FOOD REACTION TRACKER

Use this tracker to monitor your reactions to certain foods or download your free food journal at TerriWard.com/journal-food-mood-poop-download.

	FOODS EATEN	BOWEL MOVEMENT?	ABDOMINAL PAIN (1–10)	FLARE-UP?
SUN				
MON				
TUE				
WED				
THUR				
FRI				
SAT				

STRESS & EMOTIONS	NAUSEA? VOMITING? DIARRHEA? CONSTIPATION?	OTHER NOTES

RESOURCES

Ingredients and Supplements

Alternative Flour, Pastas, and More

BobsRedMill.com

ThriveMarket.com

Amazon.com

I recommend these online sources for purchasing alternative flours, starches, gluten-free grits, and other pantry items like lentil and chickpea pastas.

Diverticulitis Tea

CalmingBlends.com

This tea contains organic chamomile, peppermint, marshmallow leaves, and wild yam root and has antispasmodic properties to help reduce intestinal spasms and cramping.

Electrolytes

UltimaReplenisher.com

DrinkLMNT.com

TraceMinerals.com

DesignsforHealth.com

These sites sell electrolytes without sugar, gluten, and artificial ingredients.

Licorice Root Tea

TraditionalMedicinals.com

Anti-inflammatory licorice root has been used in herbal medicine for centuries to treat gastrointestinal distress. This licorice root tea is naturally sweet and soothing. It can also be found on Amazon.

Liquid Multivitamins

QuicksilverScientific.com

MaryRuthOrganics.com

DesignsforHealth.com

Pills can be problematic when digestion is compromised. Liquid vitamins can be more digestible, bioavailable, and absorbable.

Magnesium

NaturalVitality.com

JigsawHealth.com

Magnesium acts as a laxative by relaxing your intestinal muscles and pulling water in to make stool softer and easier to move. Natural Vitality's Calm provides magnesium citrate in a powder, and Jigsaw Health's MagSRT is a sustained-release magnesium tablet.

Psyllium Husk Powder, Wakame, and Herbs

MountainRoseHerbs.com

This site is where you can find psyllium husk, wakame, hibiscus, and gut-healing herbs like marshmallow root, slippery elm, and licorice root. You might also find psyllium husk in the pharmacy section of your grocery store.

UltraInflamXPlus 360°

Metagenics.com

This vegan medical food has gut-healing, anti-inflammatory ingredients formulated to provide nutritional support for compromised gut function.

Recommended Reading

Bristol Stool Chart

Health.com/condition/digestive-health/bristol-stool-chart

This article includes the Bristol Stool chart to help you identify what a healthy stool looks like so you know what to aim for and what other shapes might mean.

Soaking and Sprouting Nuts

Draxe.com/nutrition/sprout

This article explains the why and how for soaking and sprouting nuts, grains, beans, and seeds.

Tools and Equipment

Fermenting

CulturesforHealth.com

Cultures for Health has helpful information and supplies for fermenting. Amazon.com also has airlock lids, fermenting weights, and plastic mason jar lids.

Oil Infusion

Extension.PSU.edu/how-to-safely-make-infused-oils

Use this helpful resource to learn how to acidify and infuse oils for shelf-stability.

Popsicle Bags

Amazon.com

Popsicle bags are a convenient alternative to popsicle molds. Look for BPA-free bags.

Squatty Potty

SquattyPotty.com

Squatty Potty puts your body in a natural, comfy squat to properly align your colon for an easier and more complete elimination.

REFERENCES

American Gastroenterological Association. "Management of Acute Diverticulitis Guideline Patient Companion." Accessed February 7, 2022. gastro.org/guidelines/liver-diseases/management-of-acute-diverticulitis.

Böhm SK. "Risk Factors for Diverticulosis, Diverticulitis, Diverticular Perforation, and Bleeding: A Plea for More Subtle History Taking." *Viszeralmedizin: Gastrointestinal Medicine and Surgery.* 2015; 31(2): 84–94. doi:10.1159/000381867.

Boynton W, Floch M. "New Strategies for the Management of Diverticular Disease: Insights for the Clinician." *Therapeutic Advances in Gastroenterology.* 2013; 6(3): 205–213. doi:10.1177/1756283X13478679.

Carabotti M, Falangone F, Cuomo R, Annibale B. "Role of Dietary Habits in the Prevention of Diverticular Disease Complications: A Systematic Review." *Nutrients.* 2021; 13(4). doi:10.3390/nu13041288.

Chabok A, Påhlman L, Hjern F, Haapaniemi S, Smedh K. "Randomized Clinical Trial of Antibiotics in Acute Uncomplicated Diverticulitis." *British Journal of Surgery.* 2012; 99(4): 532–539. doi:10.1002/bjs.8688.

Cleveland Clinic. "Diverticulosis and Diverticulitis of the Colon." Accessed February 7, 2022. my.clevelandclinic.org/health/diseases/10352 -diverticular-disease.

Daniels L, Unlü Ç, de Korte N, et al. "Randomized Clinical Trial of Observational versus Antibiotic Treatment for a First Episode of CT-Proven Uncomplicated Acute Diverticulitis." *British Journal of Surgery.* 2017; 104(1): 52–61. doi:10.1002/bjs.10309.

Hawkins AT, Wise PE, Chan T, et al. "Diverticulitis: An Update From the Age Old Paradigm." *Current Problems in Surgery.* 2020; 57(10): 100862. doi:10.1016 /j.cpsurg.2020.100862.

Morris ZS, Wooding S, Grant J. "The Answer Is 17 Years, What Is the Question: Understanding Time Lags in Translational Research." *Journal of the Royal Society of Medicine.* 2011; 104(12): 510–520. doi:10.1258/jrsm.2011.110180.

Nasef NA, Mehta S. "Role of Inflammation in Pathophysiology of Colonic Disease: An Update." *International Journal of Molecular Sciences.* 2020; 21(13): 1–22. doi:10.3390/ijms21134748.

Piscopo N, Ellul P. "Diverticular Disease: A Review on Pathophysiology and Recent Evidence." *The Ulster Medical Journal.* 2020; 89(2): 83–88.

Ticinesi A, Nouvenne A, Corrente V, Tana C, di Mario F, Meschi T. "Diverticular Disease: A Gut Microbiota Perspective." *Journal of Gastrointestinal and Liver Diseases.* 2019; 28(3): 327–337. doi:10.15403/jgld-277.

Tursi A. "Current and Evolving Concepts on the Pathogenesis of Diverticular Disease." *Journal of Gastrointestinal and Liver Diseases.* 2019; 28(2): 225–235. doi:10.15403/jgld-184.

Violi A, Cambiè G, Miraglia C, et al. "Epidemiology and Risk Factors for Diverticular Disease." *Acta Biomedica.* 2018; 89: 107–112. doi:10.23750/abm.v89i9-S.7924.

INDEX

Acknowledgments

First and foremost, I'd like to thank my husband for being my sounding board and ultimate taste-tester of all things not coconut and for putting up with research papers and recipes all over the kitchen island the past few months.

Next, I want to thank my editor, Rachelle Cihonski, for her support, diligence in getting things right, and awesome suggestions.

Thank you to Karen Dvornich, FNTP, CGP, and Andrea Crane, MS, BSN, BS, for always being there when I need technical or emotional support. I greatly appreciate their encouragement and help.

Finally, thank you to my project team at Callisto Media for all their hard work and support. It truly takes a village and so many people had important roles in getting this book published.

About the Author

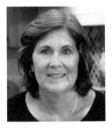 **Terri Ward, MS, FNTP, CGP,** is a functional nutritionist who started cooking and meal planning as a young child. When autoimmunity and food intolerances struck her and her family, she took charge of her health and drastically changed her diet. She upgraded her culinary skills and learned to transform recipes into healthy, allergy-friendly dishes.

Despite Terri's recipes having no gluten, dairy, or refined sugar and minimal-to-no soy, guests love her dishes and don't notice what's missing. With Terri's creativity, along with her love for food and writing, she has become a source of inspiration and encouragement to others suffering from health challenges. She shares her recipes in customized meal plans for clients and on her blog at TerriWard.com.